OWEN HUNTER

Folliculitis

Your Comprehensive Blueprint for Diagnosis and Treatment

Contents

INTRODUCTION

Folliculitis, a common skin condition characterized by the inflammation of hair follicles, affects millions of people worldwide. It can manifest as small, red, itchy, or painful bumps on the skin, often resembling acne or a rash. While folliculitis is not typically life-threatening, it can cause significant discomfort, embarrassment, and even long-term skin damage if left untreated.

Despite its prevalence, folliculitis remains a poorly understood condition among the general public. Many people struggle to identify the symptoms, causes, and appropriate treatment options, leading to frustration and a sense of helplessness. The lack of accessible, comprehensive information about folliculitis has created a gap in the market for a book that not only educates readers but also provides practical guidance and support.

This book aims to fill that gap by offering a holistic approach to understanding, managing, and living well with folliculitis. Drawing upon the latest scientific research, expert insights, and real-life experiences of individuals with folliculitis, this book is designed to be an invaluable resource for anyone seeking to navigate this challenging skin condition.

The journey begins with a thorough overview of folliculitis in Chapter 1, which delves into the different types of folliculitis, common symptoms, and risk factors. By providing a clear and concise understanding of the condition, readers will be better equipped to recognize the signs of folliculitis and take the first steps towards effective management.

Chapter 2 explores the various causes and triggers of folliculitis, ranging from bacterial, fungal, and viral infections to non-infectious factors such as lifestyle and environmental influences. Understanding the underlying causes is crucial for developing targeted prevention and treatment strategies, which will be discussed in later chapters.

Accurate diagnosis is the foundation of successful treatment, and Chapter 3 guides readers through the process of evaluation, including medical history, physical examination, laboratory tests, and skin biopsy. This chapter also touches upon the importance of differential diagnosis, as folliculitis can sometimes mimic other skin conditions.

Chapters 4 and 5 dive into the management of acute and chronic folliculitis, respectively. Acute folliculitis, characterized by sudden outbreaks, can be distressing and require prompt intervention. This book provides detailed information on dealing with superficial folliculitis, deep folliculitis, gram-negative folliculitis, and the notorious "hot tub folliculitis." Chronic folliculitis, on the other hand, demands a more long-term approach. Readers will learn about the challenges and strategies associated with persistent cases such as sycosis barbae, pseudofolliculitis barbae, eosinophilic folliculitis, and folliculitis decalvans.

Recognizing that folliculitis can affect different populations in unique ways, Chapter 6 focuses on special considerations for children, immunocompromised individuals, athletes, and people with skin of color. By addressing the specific needs and concerns of these groups, this book aims to provide targeted guidance and support.

Folliculitis can lead to various complications and related conditions, which are discussed in Chapter 7. Readers will learn about the potential for scarring, skin damage, recurrent infections, and the link between folliculitis and other skin disorders such as folliculitis keloidalis nuchae and hidradenitis suppurativa. Awareness of these complications underscores the importance of timely intervention and appropriate care.

Chapters 8 and 9 explore the array of topical and systemic therapies available for treating folliculitis. From antibacterial cleansers and topical antibiotics to oral medications and retinoids, readers will gain insights into the various options and their indications. The book also discusses the role of light and laser therapies in Chapter 10, including photodynamic therapy, pulsed dye laser, Nd:YAG laser, and intense pulsed light (IPL).

Prevention is a key aspect of managing folliculitis, and Chapter 11 offers practical strategies for minimizing the risk of flare-ups. Readers will learn about the importance of skin hygiene, hair removal techniques, clothing choices, and lifestyle modifications that can help keep folliculitis at bay.

Beyond the physical aspects of folliculitis, this book also addresses the significant impact the condition can have on quality of life. Chapter 12 delves into the psychological implications, social stigma, and self-esteem issues that often accompany folliculitis. Readers will find coping strategies, information on support groups, and guidance on communicating effectively with healthcare providers.

As research into folliculitis continues to evolve, Chapter 13 explores emerging therapies and future directions in treatment. From microbiome modulation and targeted immunotherapies to stem cell therapies and ongoing clinical trials, this chapter offers hope for individuals seeking novel approaches to managing their condition.

Finally, Chapter 14 brings together all the knowledge and insights from the previous chapters to provide a comprehensive guide to living well with folliculitis. Readers will learn how to develop personalized treatment plans, incorporate nutrition and diet for healthy skin, manage stress, and empower themselves through advocacy and education.

Throughout the book, readers will find a wealth of practical tips, real-life anecdotes, and expert advice to help them navigate the challenges of folliculitis. The appendices provide a glossary of terms, a list of resources and support organizations, and references for further reading, ensuring that readers have access to all the tools they need to take control of their skin health.

By combining cutting-edge research, holistic approaches, and a compassionate tone, this book aims to become the go-to resource for anyone affected by folliculitis. Whether you are newly diagnosed, have been struggling with the condition for years, or are supporting a loved one with folliculitis, this book will provide the knowledge, guidance, and empowerment you need to live well and thrive.

CHAPTER 1

Chapter 1: Understanding Folliculitis: An Overview

1.1 What is Folliculitis?

Folliculitis is a common skin condition that occurs when hair follicles become inflamed or infected. Hair follicles are tiny pockets in the skin from which hair grows. When these follicles are damaged or blocked, they can become susceptible to infection by bacteria, fungi, or viruses, leading to the development of folliculitis.

The term "folliculitis" comes from the Latin words "folliculus," meaning small bag or sac, and "-itis," meaning inflammation. This etymology accurately describes the condition, as folliculitis involves the inflammation of the hair follicles, which are essentially small sacs in the skin.

Folliculitis can affect people of all ages, genders, and ethnicities, although certain factors may increase the risk of developing the condition. These risk factors will be discussed in more detail later in this chapter.

1.2 Types of Folliculitis

Folliculitis can be classified into several types based on the depth of inflammation, the causative agent, and the duration of the condition. Understanding the different types of folliculitis is essential for accurate diagnosis and effective treatment.

1.2.1 Superficial Folliculitis

Superficial folliculitis involves inflammation of the upper part of the hair follicle. It is the most common type of folliculitis and is often caused by bacterial or fungal infections. Examples of superficial folliculitis include:

a. Bacterial Folliculitis: This type is caused by bacterial infections, most commonly by Staphylococcus aureus. It is characterized by small, red, itchy, or tender bumps surrounding hair follicles.

b. Pseudomonas Folliculitis (Hot Tub Folliculitis): This type is caused by the bacterium Pseudomonas aeruginosa and is often associated with exposure to contaminated water in hot tubs, swimming pools, or saunas.

c. Pityrosporum Folliculitis: This type is caused by an overgrowth of the yeast Malassezia, which normally lives on the skin. It is more common in young adults and often affects the upper back, chest, and shoulders.

1.2.2 Deep Folliculitis

Deep folliculitis involves inflammation of the entire hair follicle and the surrounding tissue. It is less common than superficial folliculitis but can be more severe and lead to scarring. Examples of deep folliculitis include:

a. Sycosis Barbae: This type affects the beard area in men and is often caused by the bacterium Staphylococcus aureus.

b. Gram-Negative Folliculitis: This type is caused by gram-negative bacteria and usually occurs in individuals who have been on long-term antibiotic treatment for acne.

c. Eosinophilic Folliculitis: This type is characterized by the presence of eosinophils, a type of white blood cell, in the inflamed follicles. It is more common in people with HIV/AIDS.

1.2.3 Chronic Folliculitis

Chronic folliculitis refers to cases where the condition persists or recurs over time. Examples of chronic folliculitis include:

a. Pseudofolliculitis Barbae: Also known as "razor bumps," this type occurs when shaved hair curls back and grows into the skin, causing inflammation. It is more common in individuals with curly hair.

b. Folliculitis Decalvans: This type is a rare form of chronic folliculitis that leads to scarring and permanent hair loss on the scalp.

1.3 Symptoms and Signs

The symptoms of folliculitis can vary depending on the type and severity of the condition. However, some common signs and symptoms include:

- Small, red, itchy, or painful bumps surrounding hair follicles
    - Pus-filled blisters or pustules
    - Tenderness or burning sensation on the affected skin
    - Swelling and redness around the hair follicles
    - Crusty or scaly skin
    - Recurrent or persistent bumps or rashes

In some cases, folliculitis can lead to complications such as scarring, hyper-pigmentation (darkening of the skin), or permanent hair loss. It is essential to seek prompt medical attention if the condition is severe, persistent, or if you experience any signs of a more serious infection, such as fever or chills.

1.4 Risk Factors

Several factors can increase the risk of developing folliculitis. These include:

1.4.1 Medical Conditions

Certain medical conditions can make individuals more susceptible to folliculitis. These include:

- Diabetes
    - HIV/AIDS
    - Chronic leukemia
    - Organ transplantation (due to immunosuppressive medications)
    - Acne or dermatitis

1.4.2 Lifestyle Factors

Lifestyle habits and environmental factors can also contribute to the development of folliculitis. These include:

- Shaving, waxing, or plucking hair
    - Wearing tight or non-breathable clothing
    - Using shared equipment at gyms or pools
    - Exposure to hot and humid environments
    - Smoking
    - Obesity

1.4.3 Medications

Some medications can increase the risk of folliculitis as a side effect. These include:

- Long-term antibiotic therapy

- Corticosteroids
- Certain acne medications (e.g., topical or oral retinoids)

1.4.4 Skin Damage or Trauma

Damage or trauma to the skin can make hair follicles more vulnerable to infection. This can occur due to:

- Abrasions or cuts
    - Excessive scratching or rubbing
    - Insect bites
    - Chemical irritants or harsh skincare products

Understanding the risk factors for folliculitis can help individuals take preventive measures and identify potential triggers for their condition. However, it is important to note that having one or more of these risk factors does not necessarily mean that a person will develop folliculitis.

In conclusion, folliculitis is a common skin condition that can cause significant discomfort and distress for those affected. By understanding the different types of folliculitis, recognizing the symptoms and signs, and being aware of the risk factors, individuals can take steps towards effective management and prevention of the condition.

This chapter has provided a comprehensive overview of folliculitis, laying the foundation for the subsequent chapters that will delve deeper into the causes, diagnosis, treatment, and management of this condition. As we move forward, it is essential to remember that folliculitis is a complex condition that requires a holistic approach, taking into account not only the physical aspects but also the psychological and social impact on an individual's quality of life.

By arming ourselves with knowledge and understanding, we can empower ourselves and others to take control of our skin health and find the best path towards healing and living well with folliculitis. The journey may not always be easy, but with the right information, support, and guidance, it is possible to manage this condition effectively and lead a fulfilling life.

In the next chapter, we will explore the various causes and triggers of folliculitis, providing valuable insights into the underlying mechanisms of this condition and paving the way for targeted prevention and treatment strategies.

CHAPTER 2

hapter 2: Causes and Triggers of Folliculitis

Folliculitis is a multifaceted skin condition that can be caused by a variety of factors, ranging from infectious agents to lifestyle habits and environmental influences. Understanding the underlying causes and triggers of folliculitis is crucial for developing effective prevention and treatment strategies. In this chapter, we will explore the various factors that can contribute to the development of folliculitis, including bacterial, fungal, and viral infections, as well as non-infectious causes and lifestyle and environmental factors.

2.1 Bacterial Infections

Bacterial infections are among the most common causes of folliculitis. The skin is home to a diverse array of bacteria, many of which are harmless or even beneficial. However, when the delicate balance of the skin's microbiome is disrupted, certain bacteria can multiply and lead to infection.

2.1.1 Staphylococcus aureus

Staphylococcus aureus, often referred to as "staph," is a common bacterium found on the skin and in the nose of many healthy individuals. However, when this bacterium enters the hair follicles through cuts, abrasions, or other damage to the skin, it can cause folliculitis. Staph folliculitis is characterized by red, swollen, and painful bumps around hair follicles, often filled with pus.

Risk factors for staph folliculitis include:

- Close contact with an infected individual
    - Sharing personal items, such as towels or razors
    - Weakened immune system
    - Skin conditions that cause breaks in the skin, such as eczema or acne

2.1.2 Pseudomonas aeruginosa

Pseudomonas aeruginosa is a bacterium that thrives in warm, moist environments. It is a common cause of "hot tub folliculitis," also known as "pseudomonas folliculitis." This type of folliculitis occurs when the bacterium enters hair follicles through contaminated water in hot tubs, swimming pools, or saunas.

Symptoms of hot tub folliculitis usually appear within 48 hours of exposure and include:

- Red, itchy, or tender bumps around hair follicles
    - Pustules or blisters
    - Rash-like appearance

To prevent hot tub folliculitis, it is essential to maintain proper hygiene and water quality in hot tubs and swimming pools.

2.1.3 Other Bacterial Causes

While Staphylococcus aureus and Pseudomonas aeruginosa are the most common bacterial causes of folliculitis, other bacteria can also contribute to the condition. These include:

- Streptococcus species
    - Enterobacteriaceae (gram-negative bacteria)
    - Propionibacterium acnes (now known as Cutibacterium acnes)

In some cases, folliculitis can be caused by a combination of different bacteria, making treatment more challenging.

2.2 Fungal Infections

Fungal infections are another common cause of folliculitis. The most prevalent fungal culprit is a yeast called Malassezia, which is a normal inhabitant of the skin.

2.2.1 Pityrosporum Folliculitis

Pityrosporum folliculitis, also known as Malassezia folliculitis, occurs when there is an overgrowth of the Malassezia yeast on the skin. This type of folliculitis is more common in young adults and often affects the upper back, chest, and shoulders.

Factors that can contribute to the development of pityrosporum folliculitis include:

- Hot and humid climates
    - Excessive sweating
    - Oily skin
    - Immunosuppression
    - Long-term antibiotic use

Symptoms of pityrosporum folliculitis include itchy, red, or inflamed bumps around hair follicles, often accompanied by a burning or stinging sensation.

2.2.2 Other Fungal Causes

While Malassezia is the most common fungal cause of folliculitis, other fungi can also lead to the condition. These include:

- Dermatophytes (e.g., Trichophyton and Microsporum species)
    - Candida species

Fungal folliculitis can be more challenging to treat than bacterial folliculitis, as antifungal medications may be required in addition to lifestyle modifications.

2.3 Viral Infections

Although less common than bacterial and fungal causes, viral infections can also contribute to the development of folliculitis.

2.3.1 Herpes Simplex Virus

Herpes simplex virus (HSV) is a common viral infection that can cause folliculitis, particularly in the genital or facial areas. HSV folliculitis is characterized by clusters of small, painful blisters or sores around hair follicles.

Risk factors for HSV folliculitis include:

- Direct contact with an infected individual
    - Weakened immune system
    - Skin damage or trauma

Treatment for HSV folliculitis typically involves antiviral medications, such as acyclovir or valacyclovir.

2.3.2 Other Viral Causes

Other viruses that can cause folliculitis include:

- Molluscum contagiosum virus
  - Varicella-zoster virus (the cause of chickenpox and shingles)

Viral folliculitis can be more difficult to diagnose and treat than bacterial or fungal folliculitis, as the symptoms may mimic other skin conditions.

2.4 Non-Infectious Causes

While infections are the most common causes of folliculitis, non-infectious factors can also contribute to the development of the condition.

2.4.1 Mechanical Irritation

Mechanical irritation of the hair follicles can lead to a type of folliculitis called "pseudofolliculitis barbae," also known as "razor bumps." This condition occurs when shaved or plucked hair curls back and grows into the skin, causing inflammation and bumps.

Pseudofolliculitis barbae is more common in individuals with curly or coarse hair, particularly in the beard area, pubic region, and legs. To prevent this type of folliculitis, it is essential to use proper hair removal techniques and avoid close shaving.

2.4.2 Chemical Irritants

Exposure to certain chemicals or harsh skincare products can irritate the hair follicles and lead to folliculitis. Examples of potential irritants include:

- Certain hair care products, such as gels or sprays
  - Skincare products containing alcohol or fragrances
  - Industrial chemicals, such as oils or solvents

To minimize the risk of chemical irritation, it is important to use gentle, non-comedogenic skincare products and avoid exposure to harsh chemicals whenever possible.

2.4.3 Occlusion

Occlusion, or the blockage of hair follicles, can contribute to the development of folliculitis. Factors that can cause occlusion include:

- Tight or non-breathable clothing
    - Prolonged sitting or pressure on the skin
    - Excessive sweating
    - Heavy, oily skincare products

To prevent occlusion-related folliculitis, it is important to wear loose, breathable clothing, maintain good hygiene, and use lightweight, non-comedogenic skincare products.

2.5 Lifestyle and Environmental Factors

In addition to the specific causes discussed above, various lifestyle and environmental factors can increase the risk of developing folliculitis or exacerbate existing symptoms.

2.5.1 Hot and Humid Environments

Hot and humid environments can create ideal conditions for the growth of bacteria and fungi on the skin, increasing the risk of folliculitis. This is particularly true for individuals who are prone to excessive sweating or those who wear tight, non-breathable clothing in these conditions.

To minimize the risk of folliculitis in hot and humid environments, it is essential to:

- Wear loose, breathable clothing
    - Use lightweight, non-comedogenic skincare products
    - Shower and change clothing after excessive sweating
    - Maintain proper hygiene in shared facilities, such as gyms or saunas

2.5.2 Smoking

Smoking has been identified as a potential risk factor for folliculitis. Cigarette smoke can irritate the skin and hair follicles, making them more susceptible to infection. Additionally, smoking can impair the immune system, making it more difficult for the body to fight off infections.

To reduce the risk of folliculitis associated with smoking, quitting or cutting back on cigarette use is strongly recommended.

2.5.3 Obesity

Obesity can increase the risk of folliculitis due to several factors, including:

- Increased sweating and moisture in skin folds
    - Friction and irritation from skin rubbing together
    - Hormonal changes that can affect the skin's microbiome

Maintaining a healthy weight through a balanced diet and regular exercise can help reduce the risk of obesity-related folliculitis.

2.5.4 Stress

Chronic stress has been linked to a variety of skin conditions, including folliculitis. Stress can weaken the immune system, making the skin more vulnerable to infections. Additionally, stress can lead to behaviors that may exacerbate folliculitis, such as picking or scratching at the skin.

Managing stress through relaxation techniques, such as meditation, deep breathing, or yoga, can help support skin health and reduce the risk of folliculitis flare-ups.

In conclusion, folliculitis can be caused by a wide range of factors, from infectious agents like bacteria, fungi, and viruses to non-infectious causes like mechanical irritation, chemical irritants, and occlusion. Lifestyle and environmental factors, such as hot and humid environments, smoking, obesity, and stress, can also contribute to the development or exacerbation of folliculitis.

By understanding the various causes and triggers of folliculitis, individuals can take proactive steps to minimize their risk of developing the condition or experiencing recurrent flare-ups. This may involve adopting healthy lifestyle habits, maintaining good hygiene, using gentle skincare products, and managing underlying medical conditions.

It is important to note that the causes and triggers of folliculitis can vary from person to person, and what may cause a flare-up in one individual may not affect another. As such, it is essential to work closely with a healthcare provider to identify the specific factors contributing to one's folliculitis and develop a personalized prevention and treatment plan.

In the next chapter, we will delve into the diagnosis and evaluation of folliculitis, exploring the various tools and techniques used by healthcare professionals to accurately identify the condition and develop effective treatment strategies. By combining the knowledge gained from this chapter on causes and triggers with the insights from the upcoming chapter on diagnosis and evaluation, readers will be well-equipped to take an informed and proactive approach to managing their folliculitis.

CHAPTER 3

hapter 3: Diagnosis and Evaluation

C Accurately diagnosing and evaluating folliculitis is crucial for developing effective treatment plans and managing the condition. In this chapter, we will explore the various tools and techniques used by healthcare professionals to identify folliculitis, determine its underlying causes, and differentiate it from other skin conditions. By understanding the diagnostic process, individuals can better advocate for their own health and work collaboratively with their healthcare providers to achieve optimal outcomes.

3.1 Medical History and Physical Examination

The first step in diagnosing folliculitis is a thorough medical history and physical examination. During this process, a healthcare provider will gather information about the patient's symptoms, onset and duration of the condition, and any potential triggers or risk factors.

3.1.1 Medical History

A comprehensive medical history will include questions about:

- The location, appearance, and severity of the affected areas
  - The duration and frequency of flare-ups

- Any associated symptoms, such as itching, pain, or discharge
- Recent exposure to potential triggers, such as hot tubs, shared equipment, or new skincare products
- Personal and family history of skin conditions or autoimmune disorders
- Current medications, including antibiotics, corticosteroids, or immuno-suppressants
- Lifestyle factors, such as smoking, diet, and stress levels

This information can help healthcare providers identify potential causes or contributing factors and guide further diagnostic tests or treatment decisions.

3.1.2 Physical Examination

During the physical examination, the healthcare provider will carefully inspect the affected areas, noting the appearance, distribution, and severity of the lesions. They may also assess the overall health and appearance of the skin, looking for signs of dryness, irritation, or other underlying skin conditions.

The physical examination can help determine the type of folliculitis (e.g., superficial or deep) and identify any complications, such as scarring or secondary infections. In some cases, the healthcare provider may use a dermatoscope, a specialized magnifying tool, to examine the hair follicles and surrounding skin more closely.

3.2 Laboratory Tests

In addition to the medical history and physical examination, laboratory tests may be necessary to confirm the diagnosis of folliculitis, identify the underlying cause, or rule out other skin conditions.

3.2.1 Bacterial Culture

If bacterial folliculitis is suspected, a bacterial culture may be performed. This involves taking a sample of the affected skin or pus from a lesion and growing it in a laboratory to identify the specific type of bacteria causing the infection. A bacterial culture can help guide antibiotic selection and determine if the infection is caused by antibiotic-resistant strains, such as methicillin-resistant Staphylococcus aureus (MRSA).

3.2.2 Fungal Culture

In cases where fungal folliculitis is suspected, a fungal culture may be necessary. Similar to a bacterial culture, a sample of the affected skin or hair is taken and grown in a laboratory to identify the specific type of fungus causing the infection. Fungal cultures can help guide antifungal treatment and rule out other conditions, such as seborrheic dermatitis or eczema.

3.2.3 Viral Testing

Although less common, viral testing may be necessary if viral folliculitis is suspected. This can involve taking a swab or scraping of the affected skin and testing it for the presence of specific viruses, such as herpes simplex virus (HSV) or molluscum contagiosum virus. Viral testing can help guide antiviral treatment and prevent the spread of the infection to others.

3.2.4 Other Laboratory Tests

Depending on the individual case and the suspected underlying causes, additional laboratory tests may be ordered, such as:

- Complete blood count (CBC) to assess overall health and rule out systemic infections
    - Metabolic panel to evaluate kidney and liver function
    - Hormonal tests to assess for conditions like polycystic ovary syndrome (PCOS) or thyroid disorders

- Inflammatory markers, such as C-reactive protein (CRP) or erythrocyte sedimentation rate (ESR), to assess for underlying inflammatory conditions

These tests can help provide a more comprehensive picture of the individual's health and guide treatment decisions.

3.3 Skin Biopsy

In some cases, a skin biopsy may be necessary to confirm the diagnosis of folliculitis or rule out other skin conditions. A skin biopsy involves removing a small sample of the affected skin for microscopic examination by a pathologist.

3.3.1 Punch Biopsy

A punch biopsy is the most common type of skin biopsy used for diagnosing folliculitis. During this procedure, the healthcare provider uses a circular tool to remove a small, cylindrical sample of skin, usually 3-4 mm in diameter. The sample is then sent to a laboratory for analysis, where a pathologist examines the tissue under a microscope to identify the presence of inflammation, infection, or other abnormalities.

3.3.2 Shave Biopsy

In some cases, a shave biopsy may be used instead of a punch biopsy. This involves using a sharp blade to remove a thin layer of skin from the affected area. Shave biopsies are generally less invasive than punch biopsies but may not provide as much information about the deeper layers of the skin.

3.3.3 Excisional Biopsy

An excisional biopsy involves removing an entire lesion or a larger area of affected skin for analysis. This type of biopsy is less commonly used for diagnosing folliculitis but may be necessary if there is concern for a more serious condition, such as skin cancer.

3.3.4 Interpreting Biopsy Results

The results of a skin biopsy can help confirm the diagnosis of folliculitis and provide information about the type and severity of the inflammation or infection. The pathologist's report may include details about the presence of bacteria, fungi, or other organisms, as well as the extent of damage to the hair follicles and surrounding skin.

Biopsy results can also help rule out other skin conditions that may mimic folliculitis, such as acne, eczema, or psoriasis. In some cases, the biopsy may reveal an underlying condition, such as lupus or sarcoidosis, that requires further evaluation and treatment.

3.4 Differential Diagnosis

Differential diagnosis is the process of distinguishing folliculitis from other skin conditions that may have similar symptoms or appearance. This is an essential step in ensuring accurate diagnosis and appropriate treatment.

3.4.1 Acne

Acne is a common skin condition that can be mistaken for folliculitis, as both involve inflammation of the hair follicles. However, acne typically affects the sebaceous glands and is characterized by the presence of comedones (blackheads and whiteheads), which are not typically seen in folliculitis. Acne lesions also tend to be more widespread and may involve the face, chest, and back, while folliculitis often occurs in localized areas.

3.4.2 Pseudofolliculitis Barbae

Pseudofolliculitis barbae, or "razor bumps," is a type of folliculitis that occurs when shaved or plucked hair curls back and grows into the skin. This condition is more common in individuals with curly or coarse hair and can be difficult to distinguish from other types of folliculitis. However, the presence of ingrown hairs and the location of the lesions (often in the beard area or on the legs) can help differentiate pseudofolliculitis barbae from other forms of folliculitis.

3.4.3 Keratosis Pilaris

Keratosis pilaris is a common skin condition characterized by small, rough, flesh-colored or red bumps that typically appear on the upper arms, thighs, or cheeks. While these bumps may resemble folliculitis, they are caused by a buildup of keratin in the hair follicles and are not typically inflamed or painful. Keratosis pilaris tends to be more widespread and symmetrical in distribution compared to folliculitis.

3.4.4 Eczema and Psoriasis

Eczema and psoriasis are chronic inflammatory skin conditions that can cause redness, scaling, and itching. In some cases, these conditions may affect the hair follicles and resemble folliculitis. However, eczema and psoriasis tend to have a more diffuse, patchy appearance and may be accompanied by other symptoms, such as dry skin or nail changes. A thorough medical history and physical examination can help differentiate these conditions from folliculitis.

3.4.5 Other Skin Conditions

Other skin conditions that may mimic folliculitis include:

- Hidradenitis suppurativa
  - Lupus erythematosus

- Sarcoidosis
- Rosacea
- Insect bites or stings
- Fungal infections, such as ringworm or tinea barbae

A thorough evaluation by a healthcare professional, along with appropriate laboratory tests and skin biopsies, can help differentiate these conditions from folliculitis and guide appropriate treatment.

In conclusion, the diagnosis and evaluation of folliculitis involve a comprehensive approach that includes a thorough medical history, physical examination, laboratory tests, and, in some cases, skin biopsies. By gathering information about the individual's symptoms, risk factors, and overall health, healthcare providers can accurately identify folliculitis and distinguish it from other skin conditions.

Accurate diagnosis is essential for developing effective treatment plans and managing the condition. In the next chapter, we will explore the various treatment options for folliculitis, including topical and systemic therapies, lifestyle modifications, and emerging treatments. By combining the knowledge gained from this chapter on diagnosis and evaluation with the insights from the upcoming chapter on treatment, individuals with folliculitis can work collaboratively with their healthcare providers to achieve optimal skin health and quality of life.

CHAPTER 4

C hapter 4: Acute Folliculitis: Dealing with Sudden Outbreaks

Acute folliculitis refers to the sudden onset of inflammation in the hair follicles, often characterized by red, itchy, or painful bumps on the skin. These outbreaks can be distressing and may require prompt treatment to alleviate symptoms and prevent complications. In this chapter, we will explore the various types of acute folliculitis, including superficial folliculitis, deep folliculitis, gram-negative folliculitis, and pseudomonas folliculitis, and discuss strategies for managing these sudden outbreaks.

4.1 Superficial Folliculitis

Superficial folliculitis is the most common type of acute folliculitis, affecting the upper part of the hair follicle. It is often caused by bacterial or fungal infections and can occur in any area of the body with hair follicles.

4.1.1 Bacterial Folliculitis

Bacterial folliculitis is typically caused by Staphylococcus aureus, a common bacterium found on the skin. When this bacterium enters the hair follicles through cuts, abrasions, or other damage to the skin, it can cause infection and inflammation.

Symptoms of bacterial folliculitis include:

- Small, red, itchy, or tender bumps around hair follicles
    - Pustules or white-headed pimples
    - Mild pain or burning sensation

Treatment for bacterial folliculitis may include:

- Topical antibiotics, such as mupirocin or clindamycin
    - Oral antibiotics, such as cephalexin or dicloxacillin, for more severe or widespread cases
    - Warm compresses to help drain pustules and reduce inflammation
    - Gentle cleansing with antibacterial soap or benzoyl peroxide wash

4.1.2 Fungal Folliculitis

Fungal folliculitis, also known as pityrosporum folliculitis, is caused by an overgrowth of the yeast Malassezia, which normally lives on the skin. This type of folliculitis is more common in young adults and often affects the upper back, chest, and shoulders.

Symptoms of fungal folliculitis include:

- Itchy, red, or inflamed bumps around hair follicles
    - Patches of small, uniform pustules
    - Burning or stinging sensation

Treatment for fungal folliculitis may include:

- Topical antifungal creams or shampoos containing ketoconazole, selenium sulfide, or pyrithione zinc
    - Oral antifungal medications, such as itraconazole or fluconazole, for severe or recurrent cases
    - Avoiding tight or non-breathable clothing
    - Using non-comedogenic and oil-free skincare products

4.2 Deep Folliculitis

Deep folliculitis involves inflammation of the entire hair follicle and the surrounding tissue. It is less common than superficial folliculitis but can be more severe and lead to scarring.

4.2.1 Furuncles and Carbuncles

Furuncles, also known as boils, are deep, painful, pus-filled bumps that develop around a hair follicle. They are usually caused by Staphylococcus aureus bacteria and can occur anywhere on the body, but are most common on the face, neck, armpits, and buttocks.

Carbuncles are clusters of interconnected furuncles that often occur in areas of friction or pressure, such as the back of the neck or thighs. They are more severe than individual furuncles and can lead to systemic symptoms like fever and fatigue.

Treatment for furuncles and carbuncles may include:

- Warm compresses to help drain the pus and reduce pain
    - Topical or oral antibiotics, depending on the severity and extent of the infection
    - Incision and drainage by a healthcare professional for large or persistent lesions
    - Pain management with over-the-counter medications like ibuprofen or acetaminophen

4.2.2 Hidradenitis Suppurativa

Hidradenitis suppurativa is a chronic, recurrent form of deep folliculitis that affects the apocrine sweat glands, primarily in the armpits, groin, and under the breasts. It is characterized by the formation of painful, inflamed nodules that can rupture and release pus, leading to scarring and sinus tract formation.

Treatment for hidradenitis suppurativa may include:

- Topical or oral antibiotics to control bacterial growth and reduce inflammation
    - Retinoids, such as isotretinoin or acitretin, to reduce sebum production and prevent follicular occlusion
    - Immunosuppressants, like adalimumab or infliximab, for severe or refractory cases
    - Surgical procedures, such as excision or laser therapy, to remove affected tissue and prevent recurrence

4.3 Gram-Negative Folliculitis

Gram-negative folliculitis is a type of acute folliculitis caused by gram-negative bacteria, such as Klebsiella, Enterobacter, or Pseudomonas species. It often occurs in individuals who have been on long-term antibiotic treatment for acne or other conditions, as the antibiotics can disrupt the normal balance of skin bacteria and allow gram-negative organisms to overgrow.

Symptoms of gram-negative folliculitis include:

- Sudden onset of red, tender, or pustular bumps around hair follicles
    - Lesions that are often more superficial than those seen in other types of folliculitis
    - Resistance to standard antibiotic treatments

Treatment for gram-negative folliculitis may include:

- Discontinuation of the current antibiotic regimen
    - Targeted antibiotics based on bacterial culture and sensitivity results

 - Topical benzoyl peroxide or chlorhexidine to reduce bacterial load on the skin
    - Oral isotretinoin for severe or recurrent cases

4.4 Pseudomonas Folliculitis (Hot Tub Folliculitis)

Pseudomonas folliculitis, also known as hot tub folliculitis, is caused by the bacterium Pseudomonas aeruginosa. This type of folliculitis often occurs after exposure to contaminated water in hot tubs, swimming pools, or saunas, where the warm, moist environment promotes bacterial growth.

Symptoms of pseudomonas folliculitis include:

- Red, itchy, or tender bumps around hair follicles, often appearing within 48 hours of exposure
    - Rash-like appearance, with lesions that are typically more widespread than in other types of folliculitis
    - Self-limiting course, with symptoms resolving within 7-10 days in most cases

Treatment for pseudomonas folliculitis may include:

- Supportive care, such as cool compresses and over-the-counter anti-itch medications
    - Topical antibiotics, like polymyxin B or bacitracin, for more severe or persistent cases
    - Oral antibiotics, such as ciprofloxacin or levofloxacin, for systemic symptoms or immunocompromised individuals
    - Proper maintenance and disinfection of hot tubs and swimming pools to prevent outbreaks

Managing Acute Folliculitis: General Principles

In addition to the specific treatments mentioned above, there are several general principles that can help manage acute folliculitis and reduce the risk of recurrence:

1. Keep the affected area clean and dry: Gently cleanse the skin with mild, non-irritating soap and pat dry. Avoid scrubbing or manipulating the lesions, as this can worsen inflammation and spread infection.

2. Avoid tight or restrictive clothing: Wear loose, breathable fabrics to minimize friction and irritation of the affected area. Natural fibers like cotton or bamboo may be more comfortable than synthetic materials.

3. Manage underlying conditions: If you have an underlying condition that increases your risk of folliculitis, such as diabetes or a weakened immune system, work with your healthcare provider to optimize management and control.

4. Practice good hygiene: Regularly wash your hands, sheets, towels, and clothing to reduce the spread of infectious agents. Avoid sharing personal items like razors, towels, or loofahs.

5. Be mindful of hair removal techniques: If you are prone to folliculitis, consider alternative hair removal methods, such as electric clippers or depilatory creams, instead of close shaving or waxing. Always use clean, sharp razors and shave in the direction of hair growth.

6. Identify and avoid triggers: Pay attention to factors that seem to trigger your folliculitis outbreaks, such as certain skincare products, clothing materials, or environmental exposures. Keeping a symptom diary may help you identify patterns and make necessary adjustments.

7. Seek professional help when needed: If your folliculitis is severe, persistent, or not responding to self-care measures, consult a healthcare provider, such as

a dermatologist. They can help determine the underlying cause, recommend appropriate treatments, and monitor for complications.

Complications and When to Seek Medical Attention

While most cases of acute folliculitis resolve with proper treatment and self-care, some complications can occur, particularly with deep or severe infections. These may include:

- Scarring or hyperpigmentation of the affected skin
    - Recurrent infections or development of chronic folliculitis
    - Spread of infection to nearby hair follicles or deeper layers of the skin
    - Systemic symptoms, such as fever, chills, or rapidly spreading redness

If you experience any of the following, seek prompt medical attention:

- Severe pain, swelling, or redness around the affected area
    - Rapidly spreading infection or the appearance of red streaks on the skin
    - Fever, chills, or other signs of systemic illness
    - Folliculitis that does not respond to self-care measures or prescribed treatments
    - Recurrent episodes of folliculitis that interfere with your daily activities or quality of life

Your healthcare provider can assess the severity of your condition, rule out potential complications, and recommend appropriate interventions, which may include oral antibiotics, drainage of abscesses, or referral to a specialist.

Preventing Acute Folliculitis

While not all cases of acute folliculitis can be prevented, taking steps to maintain healthy skin and minimize risk factors can help reduce the likelihood of developing sudden outbreaks. Some preventive strategies include:

1. Maintain good skin hygiene: Regularly cleanse your skin with gentle, non-irritating products and moisturize to keep the skin barrier intact. Avoid harsh scrubs or excessive use of exfoliants, which can damage hair follicles and increase the risk of infection.

2. Shower after sweating or swimming: Promptly cleanse your skin after activities that involve sweating or exposure to potentially contaminated water, such as hot tubs or public pools. Use clean, dry towels and avoid sitting in wet clothing for extended periods.

3. Manage existing skin conditions: If you have an underlying skin condition, such as acne or dermatitis, work with your healthcare provider to keep it well-controlled. Properly managing these conditions can help reduce the risk of secondary folliculitis.

4. Optimize your skincare routine: Choose non-comedogenic, oil-free products that are less likely to clog hair follicles. If you are prone to fungal folliculitis, consider using antifungal shampoos or creams on affected areas.

5. Be cautious with hair removal: If you are susceptible to folliculitis, take care when removing hair, especially in sensitive areas like the beard, bikini line, or underarms. Consider alternative methods, such as electric clippers or depilatory creams, and always use clean, sharp tools.

6. Boost your immune system: Maintain a healthy lifestyle by eating a balanced diet, getting regular exercise, and managing stress. A strong immune system can help your body fight off infections and reduce the risk of folliculitis.

7. Avoid sharing personal items: Do not share items that come into contact with your skin, such as towels, razors, or loofahs, as this can spread infectious

agents. If you must share equipment, such as at a gym or spa, be sure to clean and disinfect items before and after use.

By understanding the various types of acute folliculitis, their causes, and appropriate management strategies, individuals can take a proactive approach to dealing with sudden outbreaks. In the next chapter, we will explore the challenges and complexities of chronic folliculitis, including conditions like sycosis barbae, pseudofolliculitis barbae, eosinophilic folliculitis, and folliculitis decalvans. By building upon the knowledge gained from this chapter on acute folliculitis, readers will be better equipped to navigate the long-term management of this persistent skin condition.

CHAPTER 5

Chapter 5: Chronic Folliculitis: Managing Persistent Cases

Chronic folliculitis refers to cases where the inflammation of hair follicles persists or recurs over an extended period. Unlike acute folliculitis, which often resolves with prompt treatment, chronic folliculitis can be more challenging to manage and may require long-term strategies to control symptoms and prevent complications. In this chapter, we will explore several types of chronic folliculitis, including sycosis barbae, pseudofolliculitis barbae, eosinophilic folliculitis, and folliculitis decalvans, and discuss approaches to managing these persistent conditions.

5.1 Sycosis Barbae

Sycosis barbae, also known as barber's itch, is a chronic form of deep folliculitis that affects the beard area in men. It is typically caused by the bacterium Staphylococcus aureus and is characterized by persistent, painful bumps and pustules around hair follicles.

5.1.1 Symptoms and Risk Factors

Symptoms of sycosis barbae include:

- Red, tender, or painful bumps in the beard area
    - Pustules or nodules that may rupture and form crusts

- Itching or burning sensation
- Scarring or skin discoloration in severe or untreated cases

Risk factors for developing sycosis barbae include:

- Close shaving or frequent hair removal
    - Improper shaving techniques or using dirty razors
    - Weakened immune system
    - Pre-existing skin conditions, such as acne or dermatitis

5.1.2 Treatment and Management

Treatment for sycosis barbae typically involves a combination of approaches, including:

1. Topical antibiotics: Applying creams or ointments containing antibiotics, such as mupirocin or clindamycin, can help control bacterial growth and reduce inflammation.

2. Oral antibiotics: For more severe or widespread cases, oral antibiotics like dicloxacillin or cephalexin may be prescribed to address the underlying infection.

3. Adjusting hair removal techniques: Temporarily avoiding shaving or using alternative methods, such as electric clippers or depilatory creams, can help minimize irritation and allow the skin to heal.

4. Proper hygiene: Regularly cleaning the beard area with mild, non-irritating soap and using clean, sharp razors can help prevent the recurrence of sycosis barbae.

5. Addressing underlying conditions: If an underlying skin condition or weakened immune system is contributing to the development of sycosis

barbae, treating these factors can help improve overall management.

In some cases, long-term low-dose oral antibiotics or retinoids may be necessary to control persistent or frequently recurring sycosis barbae.

5.2 Pseudofolliculitis Barbae

Pseudofolliculitis barbae, commonly known as razor bumps, is a chronic form of folliculitis that occurs when curly or coarse hair curls back and grows into the skin, causing inflammation and bumps. It is more common in individuals with curly or coarse hair, particularly in the beard area, pubic region, and legs.

5.2.1 Symptoms and Risk Factors

Symptoms of pseudofolliculitis barbae include:

- Small, red, or hyperpigmented bumps around hair follicles
    - Itching, tenderness, or pain in the affected area
    - Pustules or papules that may develop secondary infections

Risk factors for developing pseudofolliculitis barbae include:

- Having curly or coarse hair
    - Close shaving or frequent hair removal
    - Improper shaving techniques or using dull razors
    - Wearing tight clothing that rubs against the skin

5.2.2 Treatment and Management

Treatment for pseudofolliculitis barbae focuses on minimizing hair removal-related trauma and allowing the skin to heal. Strategies include:

1. Modifying hair removal techniques: Using electric clippers instead of close shaving, shaving in the direction of hair growth, or using depilatory creams can help reduce the risk of hair curling back into the skin.

2. Topical treatments: Applying over-the-counter hydrocortisone creams, benzoyl peroxide, or salicylic acid can help reduce inflammation and prevent secondary infections.

3. Prescription medications: For more severe cases, topical or oral antibiotics, retinoids, or steroid creams may be prescribed to control inflammation and promote healing.

4. Laser hair removal: In some cases, laser hair removal may be recommended to permanently reduce hair growth and minimize the risk of recurrent pseudofolliculitis barbae.

5. Allowing hair to grow: If possible, letting the hair grow out for several weeks can help prevent the development of new razor bumps and allow existing lesions to heal.

Maintaining a consistent skincare routine, using non-comedogenic products, and avoiding tight clothing can also help manage pseudofolliculitis barbae and reduce the likelihood of flare-ups.

5.3 Eosinophilic Folliculitis

Eosinophilic folliculitis is a chronic form of folliculitis characterized by the presence of eosinophils, a type of white blood cell, in the inflamed hair follicles. It is more common in people with HIV/AIDS but can also occur in other immunocompromised individuals or those with certain skin conditions, such as atopic dermatitis.

5.3.1 Symptoms and Risk Factors

Symptoms of eosinophilic folliculitis include:

- Intensely itchy, red, or hyperpigmented papules and pustules around hair follicles
    - Lesions that are typically concentrated on the face, neck, upper back, and chest
    - Recurrent or persistent outbreaks

Risk factors for developing eosinophilic folliculitis include:

- HIV/AIDS, particularly in individuals with low CD4 counts
    - Other immunocompromised states, such as organ transplant recipients
    - Atopic dermatitis or other eosinophilic skin conditions

5.3.2 Treatment and Management

Treatment for eosinophilic folliculitis can be challenging and may require a multifaceted approach, including:

1. Topical corticosteroids: Applying medium to high-potency topical corticosteroids can help reduce inflammation and itching in the affected areas.

2. Oral antihistamines: Non-sedating oral antihistamines, such as cetirizine or loratadine, can help control itching and minimize scratching-related damage to the skin.

3. Oral antibiotics: In some cases, oral antibiotics like minocycline or doxycycline may be prescribed to control secondary bacterial infections and reduce inflammation.

4. Immunomodulators: Topical or oral immunomodulators, such as tacrolimus or cyclosporine, may be used to suppress the immune response

and control eosinophilic folliculitis in severe or refractory cases.

5. Antiretroviral therapy: For individuals with HIV/AIDS, optimizing antiretroviral therapy and maintaining a healthy CD4 count can help improve eosinophilic folliculitis and overall skin health.

6. Phototherapy: Ultraviolet B (UVB) or psoralen and ultraviolet A (PUVA) phototherapy may be beneficial for some patients with persistent or widespread eosinophilic folliculitis.

Maintaining a gentle skincare routine, avoiding harsh products or excessive heat exposure, and managing any underlying conditions can also help control eosinophilic folliculitis and reduce the frequency of flare-ups.

5.4 Folliculitis Decalvans

Folliculitis decalvans is a rare, chronic form of folliculitis that primarily affects the scalp and can lead to permanent hair loss and scarring. It is thought to be related to an abnormal immune response to the hair follicles, although the exact cause is not well understood.

5.4.1 Symptoms and Risk Factors

Symptoms of folliculitis decalvans include:

- Painful, red, or purulent bumps on the scalp
    - Patches of hair loss with visible scarring or skin atrophy
    - Burning, itching, or tenderness in the affected areas
    - Recurrent or progressive course

Risk factors for developing folliculitis decalvans are not well-established, but the condition may be associated with:

- Genetic predisposition or family history of the condition
  - Abnormal immune response or dysfunction
  - Bacterial overgrowth on the scalp

5.4.2 Treatment and Management

Treatment for folliculitis decalvans aims to control inflammation, prevent further hair loss, and minimize scarring. Approaches may include:

1. Oral antibiotics: Long-term oral antibiotics, such as rifampicin, clindamycin, or doxycycline, are often used to control bacterial overgrowth and reduce inflammation.

2. Topical corticosteroids: Applying high-potency topical corticosteroids to the affected areas can help suppress the immune response and control inflammation.

3. Oral retinoids: In some cases, oral retinoids like isotretinoin may be prescribed to normalize follicular keratinization and reduce the risk of new lesions.

4. Immunosuppressants: For severe or refractory cases, oral immunosuppressants such as cyclosporine or mycophenolate mofetil may be considered to control the abnormal immune response.

5. Surgical interventions: In advanced cases with extensive scarring, surgical procedures like scalp reduction or hair transplantation may be necessary to improve cosmetic appearance.

6. Lifestyle modifications: Avoiding harsh hair care practices, minimizing heat styling, and using gentle, non-irritating hair products can help reduce further damage to the hair follicles.

Regular follow-up with a dermatologist is essential for monitoring the progress of folliculitis decalvans and adjusting treatment as needed. Emotional support and counseling may also be beneficial for individuals dealing with the psychosocial impact of hair loss and scarring.

Managing Chronic Folliculitis: General Principles

In addition to the specific strategies mentioned for each type of chronic folliculitis, there are several general principles that can help manage these persistent conditions:

1. Identify and address triggers: Keep a symptom diary to help identify factors that seem to trigger or worsen your folliculitis, such as certain hair removal methods, skincare products, or clothing materials. Making necessary adjustments can help reduce flare-ups.

2. Maintain a gentle skincare routine: Use mild, non-irritating cleansers and moisturizers to keep the skin barrier healthy and minimize further irritation to the hair follicles. Avoid harsh scrubs, exfoliants, or excessive heat exposure.

3. Manage underlying conditions: If you have an underlying condition that contributes to your chronic folliculitis, such as HIV/AIDS, atopic dermatitis, or an immunocompromised state, work with your healthcare provider to optimize management and control.

4. Practice good hygiene: Regularly clean the affected areas with gentle, non-irritating products and use clean, soft towels to pat dry. Avoid sharing personal items like razors, towels, or hats to minimize the risk of secondary infections.

5. Consider alternative hair removal methods: If your chronic folliculitis is related to hair removal, explore alternative methods that may be less irritating, such as electric clippers, depilatory creams, or laser hair removal. Always

follow proper techniques and use clean tools.

6. Seek professional guidance: Work closely with a dermatologist or other healthcare provider who specializes in managing chronic skin conditions. They can provide personalized advice, monitor your progress, and adjust treatment plans as needed.

7. Be patient and persistent: Managing chronic folliculitis often requires a long-term approach and may involve trial and error to find the most effective combination of treatments. Stay committed to your management plan and communicate openly with your healthcare team about any concerns or challenges.

Coping with the Physical and Emotional Impact

Living with chronic folliculitis can be physically and emotionally challenging. The persistent discomfort, visible skin changes, and potential for scarring or hair loss can impact self-esteem and quality of life. It is essential to prioritize self-care and seek support when needed:

1. Practice stress management: Engage in activities that help you manage stress, such as deep breathing, meditation, yoga, or spending time in nature. Chronic stress can exacerbate skin conditions and make management more difficult.

2. Connect with others: Consider joining a support group or online community for individuals with chronic skin conditions. Sharing your experiences and learning from others can provide valuable insights and emotional support.

3. Focus on overall health: Maintain a balanced diet, stay hydrated, exercise regularly, and prioritize sleep. A healthy lifestyle can support skin health and improve overall well-being.

4. Be kind to yourself: Avoid negative self-talk or blame related to your skin condition. Remember that chronic folliculitis is not your fault, and you are taking proactive steps to manage it.

5. Seek professional help: If you are struggling with the emotional impact of chronic folliculitis, consider speaking with a therapist or counselor who can provide coping strategies and support.

By understanding the unique challenges of chronic folliculitis and implementing a comprehensive management approach, individuals can work towards controlling symptoms, minimizing complications, and improving their quality of life. In the next chapter, we will explore the role of special populations in folliculitis, including children, immunocompromised individuals, athletes, and people with skin of color, and discuss tailored strategies for managing the condition in these groups.

CHAPTER 6

hapter 6: Special Populations and Folliculitis

Folliculitis can affect individuals of all ages, genders, and ethnicities, but certain populations may be more susceptible to developing the condition or experience unique challenges in managing it. In this chapter, we will explore the role of special populations in folliculitis, including children, immunocompromised individuals, athletes, and people with skin of color. By understanding the specific considerations and tailored strategies for each group, we can promote more effective prevention, diagnosis, and treatment of folliculitis.

6.1 Folliculitis in Children

While folliculitis can occur in individuals of any age, children may be more vulnerable to certain types of the condition due to their developing immune systems, delicate skin, and exposure to potential triggers.

6.1.1 Common Types of Folliculitis in Children

Some of the more common types of folliculitis seen in children include:

1. Bacterial folliculitis: Caused by Staphylococcus aureus or other bacteria, this type of folliculitis can occur in children of all ages and is often associated with factors such as poor hygiene, shared towels or clothing, or minor skin

injuries.

2. Pseudomonas folliculitis: Also known as "hot tub folliculitis," this type is caused by the bacterium Pseudomonas aeruginosa and is often associated with exposure to contaminated water in swimming pools, hot tubs, or water parks.

3. Eosinophilic folliculitis: While more commonly seen in adults with HIV/AIDS, eosinophilic folliculitis can also occur in children with atopic dermatitis or other eosinophilic skin conditions.

4. Fungal folliculitis: Caused by an overgrowth of the yeast Malassezia, fungal folliculitis can occur in children, particularly those with oily skin or who live in hot, humid climates.

6.1.2 Diagnosis and Treatment Considerations

Diagnosing folliculitis in children may involve a thorough skin examination, medical history, and, in some cases, skin scrapings or biopsies to identify the underlying cause. When treating folliculitis in children, healthcare providers must consider factors such as:

1. Age and weight: Medication dosages and treatment plans may need to be adjusted based on the child's age and weight to ensure safety and effectiveness.

2. Potential side effects: Some medications used to treat folliculitis, such as oral antibiotics or retinoids, may have more pronounced side effects in children and require close monitoring.

3. Compliance and administration: Treatment plans should be practical and easy for parents or caregivers to administer, taking into account the child's ability to tolerate certain medications or applications.

4. Prevention strategies: Educating parents and children about proper hygiene, avoiding shared personal items, and recognizing potential triggers can help prevent recurrent folliculitis.

Close collaboration between pediatricians, dermatologists, and parents is essential for effectively managing folliculitis in children and promoting healthy skin development.

6.2 Folliculitis in Immunocompromised Individuals

Immunocompromised individuals, such as those with HIV/AIDS, undergoing chemotherapy, or taking immunosuppressive medications, are at a higher risk of developing folliculitis and experiencing more severe or persistent cases.

6.2.1 Increased Susceptibility and Atypical Presentations

Weakened immune systems can make it more difficult for the body to fight off infections, leading to an increased susceptibility to bacterial, fungal, and viral forms of folliculitis. Additionally, immunocompromised individuals may experience atypical presentations of folliculitis, such as:

1. Eosinophilic folliculitis: This type of folliculitis is more common in people with HIV/AIDS, particularly those with low CD4 counts, and can be more severe and resistant to treatment.

2. Disseminated or deep folliculitis: Immunocompromised individuals may be more likely to develop widespread or deep folliculitis, which can lead to complications such as scarring or secondary infections.

3. Opportunistic infections: Weakened immune systems can allow less common or typically harmless microorganisms to cause folliculitis, leading to unusual presentations or challenging diagnostic processes.

6.2.2 Management Strategies

Managing folliculitis in immunocompromised individuals requires a multidisciplinary approach and close collaboration between dermatologists, infectious disease specialists, and other healthcare providers. Key strategies may include:

1. Optimizing underlying conditions: Ensuring that underlying conditions, such as HIV/AIDS or cancer, are well-managed and that medication regimens are optimized can help support immune function and improve folliculitis outcomes.

2. Tailored treatment plans: Treatment for folliculitis in immunocompromised individuals may involve a combination of topical and systemic therapies, such as antibiotics, antifungals, or immunomodulators, tailored to the specific type and severity of the condition.

3. Prophylactic measures: In some cases, prophylactic use of antimicrobial agents may be recommended to prevent recurrent or severe folliculitis in high-risk individuals.

4. Close monitoring: Regular follow-up and monitoring are essential for detecting potential complications, adjusting treatment plans, and providing ongoing support and education.

Immunocompromised individuals should also be counseled on the importance of maintaining good hygiene, avoiding potential triggers, and promptly reporting any new or worsening skin symptoms to their healthcare providers.

6.3 Folliculitis in Athletes

Athletes, particularly those involved in contact sports or activities that involve frequent skin-to-skin contact, are at an increased risk of developing folliculitis. Factors such as sweating, friction, and sharing of equipment can contribute to the spread of infectious agents and the development of folliculitis.

6.3.1 Common Types of Folliculitis in Athletes

Some of the more common types of folliculitis seen in athletes include:

1. Bacterial folliculitis: Staphylococcus aureus and other bacteria can spread easily through close contact or shared equipment, leading to outbreaks of folliculitis among teammates.

2. Pseudomonas folliculitis: Athletes who use hot tubs, whirlpools, or swimming pools that are not properly maintained may be at risk for pseudomonas folliculitis.

3. Mechanical folliculitis: Friction from tight-fitting clothing, protective gear, or equipment can lead to irritation and inflammation of hair follicles, particularly in areas like the thighs, buttocks, or underarms.

6.3.2 Prevention and Management Strategies

Preventing and managing folliculitis in athletes requires a proactive approach that involves education, hygiene, and prompt treatment. Key strategies include:

1. Proper hygiene: Athletes should be encouraged to shower immediately after practices or games, use clean towels and clothing, and avoid sharing personal items like razors or towels.

2. Equipment maintenance: Ensuring that shared equipment, such as mats or protective gear, is regularly cleaned and disinfected can help reduce the spread of infectious agents.

3. Prompt treatment: Athletes should be encouraged to report any signs of folliculitis to their trainers or healthcare providers promptly to ensure early diagnosis and treatment.

4. Modifications for active folliculitis: Athletes with active folliculitis may need to modify their training or competition schedules to allow for proper treatment and healing, and to minimize the risk of spreading the infection to others.

5. Prophylactic measures: In some cases, prophylactic use of topical antimicrobial agents may be recommended for athletes at high risk of developing folliculitis.

Coaches, trainers, and healthcare providers should work together to create a culture of open communication and proactive skin health management to minimize the impact of folliculitis on individual athletes and team performance.

6.4 Folliculitis and Skin of Color

While folliculitis can affect individuals of all skin types, people with skin of color may face unique challenges in diagnosis, treatment, and management of the condition.

6.4.1 Diagnostic Challenges

Folliculitis can present differently on darker skin tones, making it more challenging to diagnose and distinguish from other skin conditions. Some specific challenges include:

1. Hyperpigmentation: Post-inflammatory hyperpigmentation, or darkening of the skin in areas of previous inflammation, can be more pronounced in people with skin of color and may obscure the underlying folliculitis.

2. Keloid scarring: Individuals with skin of color are more prone to developing keloid scars, which are raised, firm, and often itchy or painful. Folliculitis, particularly deep or recurrent cases, can increase the risk of keloid scar formation.

3. Atypical presentations: Folliculitis may present with less visible redness or inflammation on darker skin, leading to delayed diagnosis or misdiagnosis.

6.4.2 Treatment Considerations

When treating folliculitis in people with skin of color, healthcare providers must consider potential side effects and long-term impacts on skin appearance. Some specific considerations include:

1. Hyperpigmentation: Certain topical treatments, such as benzoyl peroxide or retinoids, may cause temporary lightening or darkening of the skin, which can be more noticeable on darker skin tones.

2. Keloid scarring: Treatment plans should aim to minimize inflammation and prevent scarring, as keloids can be difficult to treat and may require additional interventions, such as intralesional corticosteroids or surgical removal.

3. Gentle skincare: People with skin of color may be more prone to irritation or sensitivity, so gentle, non-comedogenic skincare products should be recommended to avoid further inflammation.

4. Sun protection: Hyperpigmentation can be exacerbated by sun exposure, so individuals with skin of color should be counseled on the importance of using broad-spectrum sunscreen and protective clothing.

6.4.3 Cultural and Social Considerations

Healthcare providers should also be aware of cultural and social factors that may impact the management of folliculitis in people with skin of color. Some considerations include:

1. Hair care practices: Certain hair care practices, such as braiding, weaving, or using heavy oils or pomades, may increase the risk of folliculitis. Providers should discuss alternative styling methods or products that minimize irritation.

2. Skin color bias: Historical biases and lack of diversity in dermatological training and research can lead to underdiagnosis or misdiagnosis of skin conditions in people of color. Providers should actively work to recognize and address these biases in their practice.

3. Access to care: Socioeconomic disparities and lack of access to dermatological care can impact the diagnosis and management of folliculitis in communities of color. Providers should strive to create inclusive, accessible, and culturally sensitive care environments.

By understanding the unique challenges and considerations for folliculitis in people with skin of color, healthcare providers can work to improve diagnostic accuracy, treatment outcomes, and overall skin health equity.

Conclusion

Folliculitis is a complex skin condition that can affect individuals of all ages, genders, and ethnicities, but certain populations may face unique challenges in diagnosis, treatment, and management. Children, immunocompromised individuals, athletes, and people with skin of color each require tailored approaches that consider their specific needs and risk factors.

By recognizing the special considerations for each population, healthcare providers can work to develop more targeted prevention strategies, diagnostic tools, and treatment plans. This may involve collaboration between different specialties, such as pediatrics, dermatology, infectious disease, and sports medicine, to ensure comprehensive and coordinated care.

Equally important is the need for patient education and empowerment. By providing clear, culturally sensitive information about folliculitis risk factors, prevention strategies, and treatment options, healthcare providers can help individuals in these special populations take an active role in managing their skin health.

As we continue to advance our understanding of folliculitis and its impact on different populations, it is crucial that we prioritize research, education, and clinical practices that promote health equity and improve outcomes for all individuals affected by this condition.

In the next chapter, we will explore the potential complications and related conditions associated with folliculitis, highlighting the importance of prompt diagnosis and appropriate management in preventing long-term skin damage and promoting overall skin health.

CHAPTER 7

C hapter 7: Complications and Related Conditions

Folliculitis, when left untreated or ineffectively managed, can lead to various complications and related conditions that may cause significant discomfort, scarring, and emotional distress. Understanding these potential complications and their implications is crucial for both healthcare providers and individuals affected by folliculitis, as it underscores the importance of prompt diagnosis, appropriate treatment, and ongoing management. In this chapter, we will explore the main complications and related conditions associated with folliculitis, including scarring, skin damage, recurrent infections, folliculitis keloidalis nuchae, and hidradenitis suppurativa.

7.1 Scarring and Skin Damage

Scarring and skin damage are among the most common and distressing complications of folliculitis, particularly in cases of deep or recurrent infections. When the inflammation of hair follicles extends into the deeper layers of the skin, it can lead to the destruction of hair follicles and surrounding tissue, resulting in permanent scarring.

7.1.1 Types of Scarring

Folliculitis-related scarring can manifest in different forms, depending on the severity and location of the inflammation. Some common types of scarring include:

1. Atrophic scars: These scars appear as depressions in the skin and are often associated with conditions like folliculitis decalvans, which primarily affects the scalp. Atrophic scars result from the loss of collagen and elastin in the skin due to inflammation.

2. Hypertrophic scars: These scars are raised and firm, but do not extend beyond the original borders of the wound. They are more common in areas of high tension, such as the chest, back, or shoulders, and may be itchy or painful.

3. Keloid scars: Keloids are raised, firm, and often larger than the original wound. They can be itchy, painful, or tender to the touch and are more common in individuals with darker skin tones. Keloids can develop after deep or recurrent folliculitis, particularly in areas like the beard, chest, or back.

7.1.2 Pigmentation Changes

In addition to scarring, folliculitis can also lead to pigmentation changes in the affected areas. Post-inflammatory hyperpigmentation (PIH) is a common complication, especially in individuals with skin of color. PIH appears as darkened patches or spots on the skin and can persist long after the initial inflammation has resolved. In some cases, folliculitis can also cause hypopigmentation, or lightening of the skin, particularly if aggressive treatments or procedures are used.

7.1.3 Prevention and Management

Preventing scarring and skin damage from folliculitis involves prompt diagnosis and effective treatment of the underlying condition. Some strategies to minimize the risk of scarring include:

1. Early intervention: Treating folliculitis in its early stages can help prevent the inflammation from extending into the deeper layers of the skin and causing permanent damage.

2. Appropriate treatment: Using targeted therapies, such as topical or oral antibiotics, antifungals, or anti-inflammatory agents, can help control the infection and reduce the risk of scarring.

3. Gentle skincare: Avoiding picking, squeezing, or manipulating folliculitis lesions can help prevent further injury to the skin and reduce the likelihood of scarring.

4. Sun protection: Using broad-spectrum sunscreen and protective clothing can help prevent hyperpigmentation and minimize the appearance of scars.

If scarring does occur, various treatment options can help improve the appearance and texture of the skin. These may include:

1. Topical treatments: Retinoids, vitamin C, or hydroquinone can help fade hyperpigmentation and improve skin texture.

2. Intralesional corticosteroids: Injecting corticosteroids directly into hypertrophic or keloid scars can help flatten and soften them over time.

3. Laser therapy: Different types of laser treatments, such as fractional or pulsed dye lasers, can help improve the appearance of scars and even out skin tone.

4. Surgical revision: In some cases, surgical procedures may be necessary to remove or reshape severe scars.

A dermatologist or plastic surgeon can help determine the most appropriate treatment approach based on the type and severity of scarring, as well as individual patient factors.

7.2 Recurrent Infections

Recurrent infections are another potential complication of folliculitis, particularly in cases where the underlying cause is not effectively addressed or the individual has predisposing factors that increase their susceptibility.

7.2.1 Factors Contributing to Recurrent Infections

Several factors can contribute to the development of recurrent folliculitis, including:

1. Inadequate treatment: If the initial folliculitis infection is not treated with the appropriate antimicrobial agent or for a sufficient duration, the infection may not be fully eradicated, leading to recurrent episodes.

2. Antibiotic resistance: The overuse or misuse of antibiotics can lead to the development of antibiotic-resistant strains of bacteria, making subsequent infections more challenging to treat.

3. Underlying medical conditions: Certain medical conditions, such as diabetes, HIV/AIDS, or other immunocompromising disorders, can increase an individual's susceptibility to recurrent folliculitis.

4. Lifestyle factors: Factors such as excessive sweating, friction from tight clothing, or poor hygiene can create an environment that promotes the growth of bacteria and fungi, leading to recurrent infections.

5. Genetic predisposition: Some individuals may have a genetic predisposition to developing folliculitis, which can manifest as recurrent episodes or

more severe infections.

7.2.2 Management of Recurrent Infections

Managing recurrent folliculitis requires a comprehensive approach that addresses both the immediate infection and the underlying predisposing factors. Some strategies to manage recurrent infections include:

1. Culture-directed therapy: Obtaining bacterial or fungal cultures from the affected areas can help identify the specific pathogen causing the infection and guide the selection of targeted antimicrobial therapy.

2. Extended treatment courses: In some cases, longer courses of antibiotics or antifungals may be necessary to fully eradicate the infection and prevent recurrence.

3. Prophylactic therapy: For individuals with frequent recurrences, low-dose prophylactic antibiotics or topical antimicrobial agents may be recommended to prevent future infections.

4. Lifestyle modifications: Addressing predisposing factors, such as improving hygiene, wearing breathable clothing, or managing underlying medical conditions, can help reduce the risk of recurrent infections.

5. Immunomodulatory agents: In some cases, medications that modulate the immune system, such as low-dose isotretinoin or dapsone, may be used to control recurrent folliculitis.

Regular follow-up with a dermatologist is essential for monitoring the effectiveness of treatment and making necessary adjustments to prevent recurrent infections.

7.3 Folliculitis Keloidalis Nuchae

Folliculitis keloidalis nuchae (FKN), also known as acne keloidalis nuchae, is a chronic, inflammatory condition that primarily affects the hair follicles on the back of the neck and occipital scalp. While FKN is a distinct condition, it shares some features with folliculitis and can be a complication of recurrent or severe folliculitis in the affected areas.

7.3.1 Clinical Features and Risk Factors

FKN is characterized by the formation of firm, smooth, dome-shaped papules or plaques on the back of the neck or occipital scalp. These lesions can be itchy, painful, or tender and may coalesce into larger, keloidal plaques over time. In advanced cases, FKN can lead to scarring alopecia and significant cosmetic disfigurement.

Risk factors for developing FKN include:

1. Male gender: FKN is more common in men, particularly those of African or Asian descent.

2. Close shaving or haircuts: Frequent shaving or close haircuts can cause irritation and inflammation of the hair follicles, increasing the risk of FKN.

3. Friction or trauma: Rubbing or irritation from clothing, helmets, or other headgear can contribute to the development of FKN.

4. Genetic predisposition: A family history of FKN or keloid formation may increase an individual's risk of developing the condition.

7.3.2 Management of Folliculitis Keloidalis Nuchae

Managing FKN can be challenging, as the condition tends to be chronic and recurrent. Treatment options may include:

1. Topical therapies: Corticosteroids, retinoids, or antimicrobial agents can help reduce inflammation and prevent secondary infections.

2. Intralesional corticosteroids: Injecting corticosteroids directly into the FKN lesions can help soften and flatten the keloidal plaques.

3. Oral medications: Antibiotics, isotretinoin, or immunomodulatory agents may be used to control inflammation and prevent progression of the condition.

4. Laser therapy: Laser hair removal or ablative laser resurfacing can help reduce the risk of recurrent folliculitis and improve the appearance of FKN scars.

5. Surgical excision: In severe cases, surgical removal of the affected skin and surrounding hair follicles may be necessary to control the condition and prevent further scarring.

Prevention strategies, such as avoiding close shaving, minimizing friction or trauma to the affected areas, and maintaining good skincare habits, can help reduce the risk of developing FKN or experiencing recurrent episodes.

7.4 Hidradenitis Suppurativa

Hidradenitis suppurativa (HS), also known as acne inversa, is a chronic, inflammatory skin condition that affects the apocrine sweat glands and surrounding hair follicles. While HS is a distinct entity, it shares some features with folliculitis and can be associated with or exacerbated by follicular inflammation.

7.4.1 Clinical Features and Risk Factors

HS is characterized by the formation of painful, inflamed nodules or abscesses in the skin folds, such as the axillae, groin, buttocks, and under the breasts. These lesions can rupture, draining pus and leading to the formation of sinus tracts and scarring. HS can have a significant impact on an individual's quality of life, causing pain, embarrassment, and disability.

Risk factors for developing HS include:

1. Genetic predisposition: A family history of HS increases an individual's risk of developing the condition.

2. Hormonal factors: HS is more common in women and may be influenced by hormonal changes, such as those associated with menstruation or pregnancy.

3. Obesity: Being overweight or obese can increase the risk of developing HS and exacerbate the severity of the condition.

4. Smoking: Cigarette smoking has been strongly associated with the development and progression of HS.

5. Mechanical friction: Friction from tight clothing or skin rubbing together can contribute to the development of HS lesions.

7.4.2 Management of Hidradenitis Suppurativa

Managing HS requires a multidisciplinary approach that addresses both the physical and psychosocial aspects of the condition. Treatment options may include:

1. Topical therapies: Antimicrobial washes, topical antibiotics, or retinoids can help control superficial inflammation and prevent secondary infections.

2. Oral medications: Antibiotics, retinoids, or immunomodulatory agents,

such as adalimumab or infliximab, may be used to control inflammation and reduce the severity of HS lesions.

3. Surgical interventions: Incision and drainage, deroofing, or wide excision of HS lesions may be necessary to control the condition and prevent recurrent infections or scarring.

4. Laser therapy: Laser hair removal or carbon dioxide laser ablation can help reduce the frequency and severity of HS flares.

5. Lifestyle modifications: Losing weight, quitting smoking, and wearing loose, breathable clothing can help minimize friction and reduce the risk of HS exacerbations.

Ongoing support and education are essential for helping individuals with HS manage their condition and maintain their quality of life. Dermatologists, plastic surgeons, and mental health professionals can work together to provide comprehensive care and support for those affected by HS.

Conclusion

Folliculitis can lead to various complications and related conditions, including scarring, skin damage, recurrent infections, folliculitis keloidalis nuchae, and hidradenitis suppurativa. These complications can cause significant physical discomfort, emotional distress, and impact an individual's quality of life. Understanding the potential consequences of untreated or poorly managed folliculitis underscores the importance of prompt diagnosis, appropriate treatment, and ongoing management.

Healthcare providers play a crucial role in helping individuals with folliculitis navigate these complications and related conditions. By recognizing the early signs of complications, initiating targeted therapies, and providing ongoing support and education, providers can help minimize the risk of long-term skin damage and improve outcomes for those affected by folliculitis.

Individuals with folliculitis can also take proactive steps to reduce their risk of complications by adhering to treatment plans, practicing good skincare habits, and making necessary lifestyle modifications. Seeking prompt medical attention for persistent or worsening symptoms and maintaining open communication with healthcare providers can help ensure timely intervention and prevent the progression of complications.

As we move forward in our understanding of folliculitis and its associated complications, ongoing research and collaboration among dermatologists, primary care providers, and other specialists will be essential for developing more effective prevention and treatment strategies. By prioritizing early intervention, patient education, and comprehensive care, we can work towards reducing the burden of folliculitis-related complications and improving the overall skin health and well-being of those affected by this condition.

In the following chapter, we will explore the various topical treatments available for folliculitis, including antibacterial cleansers, topical antibiotics, antifungal agents, and keratolytic agents. By understanding the role of these treatments in managing folliculitis and its complications, readers will be better equipped to make informed decisions about their care and work collaboratively with their healthcare providers to achieve optimal outcomes.

CHAPTER 8

hapter 8: Topical Treatments for Folliculitis

Topical treatments are a cornerstone of folliculitis management, offering targeted therapy directly to the affected skin. These treatments can help control inflammation, eradicate infectious agents, and promote healing of the hair follicles. In this chapter, we will explore the various topical treatment options for folliculitis, including antibacterial cleansers and soaps, topical antibiotics, antifungal creams and lotions, and keratolytic agents. By understanding the role of these treatments and their appropriate use, individuals with folliculitis can work with their healthcare providers to develop effective management plans and achieve optimal skin health.

8.1 Antibacterial Cleansers and Soaps

Antibacterial cleansers and soaps are often the first line of defense against folliculitis, particularly for mild to moderate cases caused by bacterial infections. These products work by reducing the number of bacteria on the skin's surface, helping to prevent the spread of infection and promote healing.

8.1.1 Types of Antibacterial Cleansers and Soaps

There are several types of antibacterial cleansers and soaps available, each with different active ingredients and mechanisms of action. Some common types include:

1. Benzoyl peroxide: Benzoyl peroxide is a topical antiseptic that works by releasing oxygen into the skin, which kills bacteria and helps unclog hair follicles. It is available in various concentrations, ranging from 2.5% to 10%, and can be found in cleansers, gels, and lotions.

2. Chlorhexidine: Chlorhexidine is a broad-spectrum antiseptic that disrupts bacterial cell membranes, leading to cell death. It is often used in surgical scrubs and is available in cleansers and wipes for folliculitis treatment.

3. Triclosan: Triclosan is an antibacterial agent that inhibits bacterial fatty acid synthesis, preventing bacterial growth and reproduction. While it was previously used in many antibacterial soaps and body washes, concerns about its safety and effectiveness have led to its removal from most consumer products.

4. Tea tree oil: Tea tree oil is a natural antiseptic derived from the leaves of the Melaleuca alternifolia tree. It has antimicrobial properties and can be found in some natural or organic skincare products, though its effectiveness may be more limited compared to other antibacterial agents.

8.1.2 Proper Use and Precautions

When using antibacterial cleansers and soaps for folliculitis, it is essential to follow proper techniques and take necessary precautions to avoid irritation or further damage to the skin. Some tips for proper use include:

1. Gently cleanse the affected areas: Use your fingertips to apply the cleanser or soap to the skin, using gentle circular motions. Avoid scrubbing or using abrasive tools, which can irritate the hair follicles.

2. Rinse thoroughly: Make sure to rinse the skin thoroughly with lukewarm water to remove all traces of the cleanser or soap.

3. Pat dry: Use a clean, soft towel to pat the skin dry, avoiding rubbing or friction.

4. Moisturize: Apply a non-comedogenic moisturizer to help maintain the skin's barrier function and prevent dryness or irritation.

Precautions to keep in mind when using antibacterial cleansers and soaps include:

1. Potential for irritation: Some antibacterial agents, such as benzoyl peroxide, can cause dryness, redness, or peeling of the skin. Start with lower concentrations and gradually increase as tolerated.

2. Allergic reactions: In rare cases, individuals may experience allergic reactions to certain antibacterial agents. If you notice any signs of an allergic reaction, such as itching, swelling, or difficulty breathing, discontinue use and seek medical attention.

3. Resistance concerns: Overuse or misuse of antibacterial agents can contribute to the development of antibiotic-resistant bacteria. Use these products as directed and only for the recommended duration.

Regular use of antibacterial cleansers and soaps, in combination with other appropriate treatments and lifestyle modifications, can help control mild to moderate folliculitis and prevent recurrent infections.

8.2 Topical Antibiotics

Topical antibiotics are another essential tool in the management of folliculitis, particularly for cases caused by bacterial infections. These medications work by killing or inhibiting the growth of bacteria directly on the skin, helping to clear infections and reduce inflammation.

8.2.1 Types of Topical Antibiotics

There are several types of topical antibiotics used for treating folliculitis, each with different mechanisms of action and spectrums of activity. Some common topical antibiotics include:

1. Clindamycin: Clindamycin is a lincosamide antibiotic that inhibits bacterial protein synthesis, leading to cell death. It is effective against a range of gram-positive bacteria, including Staphylococcus aureus, and is available in creams, gels, and lotions.

2. Erythromycin: Erythromycin is a macrolide antibiotic that also inhibits bacterial protein synthesis. It has a similar spectrum of activity to clindamycin and is available in various topical formulations.

3. Mupirocin: Mupirocin is a unique antibiotic that inhibits bacterial isoleucyl-tRNA synthetase, preventing protein synthesis. It is highly effective against Staphylococcus aureus and is often used for nasal decolonization and treatment of localized skin infections.

4. Gentamicin: Gentamicin is an aminoglycoside antibiotic that inhibits bacterial protein synthesis by binding to the 30S ribosomal subunit. It has a broad spectrum of activity, including against gram-negative bacteria, and is available in creams and ointments.

8.2.2 Proper Use and Precautions

When using topical antibiotics for folliculitis, it is crucial to follow the prescribed regimen and take necessary precautions to ensure effective treatment and minimize the risk of adverse effects or antibiotic resistance.

Some tips for proper use include:

1. Apply to clean, dry skin: Before applying the topical antibiotic, cleanse the affected area with a gentle cleanser and pat dry.

2. Use the appropriate amount: Apply a thin layer of the medication to the affected area, as directed by your healthcare provider or the product instructions.

3. Avoid contact with eyes and mucous membranes: Take care to avoid applying the medication to the eyes, nose, or mouth, as this can cause irritation or other adverse effects.

4. Wash hands after application: To prevent the spread of the medication to other parts of the body or to other people, wash your hands thoroughly with soap and water after applying the topical antibiotic.

Precautions to keep in mind when using topical antibiotics include:

1. Potential for allergic reactions: Some individuals may experience allergic reactions to certain topical antibiotics, manifesting as itching, redness, or swelling of the skin. If you suspect an allergic reaction, discontinue use and consult your healthcare provider.

2. Antibiotic resistance: Overuse or misuse of topical antibiotics can contribute to the development of antibiotic-resistant bacteria. Use these medications only as prescribed and for the recommended duration.

3. Interactions with other medications: Some topical antibiotics may interact with other medications, such as oral antibiotics or topical corticosteroids. Inform your healthcare provider of all medications you are taking before starting treatment with topical antibiotics.

Regular use of topical antibiotics, in combination with appropriate cleansing and lifestyle modifications, can effectively treat bacterial folliculitis and prevent recurrent infections. However, it is essential to follow your healthcare provider's guidance and monitor for any signs of adverse effects or treatment failure.

8.3 Antifungal Creams and Lotions

Antifungal creams and lotions are essential for treating folliculitis caused by fungal infections, such as Malassezia folliculitis or dermatophyte infections. These medications work by inhibiting the growth of fungal cells or disrupting their cell membranes, leading to cell death and clearance of the infection.

8.3.1 Types of Antifungal Creams and Lotions

There are several types of antifungal creams and lotions available for treating fungal folliculitis, each with different active ingredients and spectrums of activity. Some common antifungal agents used in topical formulations include:

1. Ketoconazole: Ketoconazole is an azole antifungal that inhibits the synthesis of ergosterol, a key component of fungal cell membranes. It is effective against a wide range of fungal species, including Malassezia and dermatophytes, and is available in creams and shampoos.

2. Clotrimazole: Clotrimazole is another azole antifungal with a similar mechanism of action to ketoconazole. It is effective against various fungal species and is commonly used in creams and lotions for treating superficial fungal infections.

3. Terbinafine: Terbinafine is an allylamine antifungal that inhibits the enzyme squalene epoxidase, disrupting fungal cell membrane synthesis. It has a particularly strong activity against dermatophytes and is available in

creams and sprays.

4. Ciclopirox: Ciclopirox is a hydroxypyridone antifungal that interferes with fungal cell membrane transport and intracellular enzyme activity. It has a broad spectrum of activity and is available in creams, lotions, and shampoos.

8.3.2 Proper Use and Precautions

When using antifungal creams and lotions for folliculitis, it is important to follow the prescribed regimen and take necessary precautions to ensure effective treatment and minimize the risk of adverse effects or treatment failure. Some tips for proper use include:

1. Apply to clean, dry skin: Before applying the antifungal cream or lotion, cleanse the affected area with a gentle cleanser and pat dry.

2. Use the appropriate amount: Apply a thin layer of the medication to the affected area, as directed by your healthcare provider or the product instructions. Some antifungal creams may require more generous application for optimal efficacy.

3. Massage gently: Gently massage the cream or lotion into the skin until it is fully absorbed, taking care not to further irritate the hair follicles.

4. Allow time for absorption: Wait a few minutes after application before dressing or applying other skincare products to allow the medication to be fully absorbed into the skin.

Precautions to keep in mind when using antifungal creams and lotions include:

1. Potential for skin irritation: Some antifungal agents, particularly those in higher concentrations, can cause skin irritation, redness, or dryness. If

you experience significant discomfort, discontinue use and consult your healthcare provider.

2. Allergic reactions: In rare cases, individuals may experience allergic reactions to certain antifungal agents, manifesting as itching, swelling, or difficulty breathing. If you suspect an allergic reaction, discontinue use and seek medical attention.

3. Interactions with other medications: Some antifungal creams and lotions may interact with other topical or systemic medications. Inform your healthcare provider of all medications you are taking before starting treatment with antifungal agents.

Consistent use of antifungal creams and lotions, in combination with appropriate cleansing and lifestyle modifications, can effectively treat fungal folliculitis and prevent recurrent infections. However, it is crucial to follow your healthcare provider's guidance and monitor for any signs of treatment failure or adverse effects.

8.4 Keratolytic Agents

Keratolytic agents are topical medications that work by softening and dissolving the keratin in the upper layers of the skin, helping to unclog hair follicles and prevent the formation of comedones. While not specifically antimicrobial, these agents can be useful adjuncts in the treatment of folliculitis, particularly for cases associated with follicular occlusion or hyperkeratosis.

8.4.1 Types of Keratolytic Agents

There are several types of keratolytic agents used in the management of folliculitis and related conditions, each with different mechanisms of action and potential side effects. Some common keratolytic agents include:

1. Salicylic acid: Salicylic acid is a beta-hydroxy acid that works by dissolving the intercellular cement between keratinocytes, promoting exfoliation and unclogging hair follicles. It is available in various concentrations in creams, lotions, and cleansers.

2. Alpha-hydroxy acids (AHAs): AHAs, such as glycolic acid and lactic acid, work similarly to salicylic acid by promoting exfoliation and reducing follicular occlusion. They are often used in lower concentrations in over-the-counter skincare products.

3. Urea: Urea is a humectant and keratolytic agent that hydrates the skin and softens keratin, making it easier to shed. It is available in various concentrations in creams and lotions.

4. Retinoids: Topical retinoids, such as tretinoin and adapalene, work by normalizing follicular keratinization and reducing inflammation. While primarily used for acne treatment, they may be helpful for some cases of folliculitis, particularly those associated with comedonal occlusion.

8.4.2 Proper Use and Precautions

When using keratolytic agents for folliculitis, it is essential to follow the prescribed regimen and take necessary precautions to minimize the risk of skin irritation or other adverse effects. Some tips for proper use include:

1. Start with lower concentrations: Begin with lower concentrations of keratolytic agents and gradually increase as tolerated to minimize the risk of skin irritation or peeling.

2. Apply to affected areas: Apply the keratolytic agent directly to the areas affected by folliculitis, avoiding contact with eyes, mucous membranes, or broken skin.

3. Use sun protection: Some keratolytic agents, particularly retinoids, can increase skin sensitivity to sunlight. Use a broad-spectrum sunscreen with an SPF of at least 30 and protective clothing when using these products.

4. Moisturize regularly: Keratolytic agents can be drying to the skin, so it is essential to use a non-comedogenic moisturizer to maintain skin hydration and prevent excessive irritation.

Precautions to keep in mind when using keratolytic agents include:

1. Potential for skin irritation: Keratolytic agents can cause redness, peeling, or dryness of the skin, particularly when used in higher concentrations or on sensitive skin. If you experience significant irritation, discontinue use and consult your healthcare provider.

2. Photosensitivity: Some keratolytic agents, such as retinoids, can increase skin sensitivity to sunlight, leading to an increased risk of sunburn or skin damage. Always use sun protection when using these products.

3. Interactions with other medications: Keratolytic agents may interact with other topical medications, such as antibiotics or antifungals. Inform your healthcare provider of all medications you are using before starting treatment with keratolytic agents.

Judicious use of keratolytic agents, in combination with appropriate antimicrobial therapy and lifestyle modifications, can help improve the efficacy of folliculitis treatment and prevent recurrent episodes. However, it is crucial to follow your healthcare provider's guidance and monitor for any signs of skin irritation or adverse effects.

Conclusion

Topical treatments are a crucial component of folliculitis management, offering targeted therapy directly to the affected skin. Antibacterial cleansers and soaps, topical antibiotics, antifungal creams and lotions, and keratolytic agents each play a unique role in controlling inflammation, eradicating infectious agents, and promoting healing of the hair follicles.

When using topical treatments for folliculitis, it is essential to follow proper techniques, take necessary precautions, and monitor for any signs of adverse effects or treatment failure. By working closely with healthcare providers and adhering to prescribed regimens, individuals with folliculitis can effectively manage their condition and achieve optimal skin health.

As we continue to explore the various treatment options for folliculitis, it is important to remember that a comprehensive approach, incorporating both topical and systemic therapies, lifestyle modifications, and patient education, is often necessary for successful long-term management. By staying informed and proactive in their care, individuals with folliculitis can take control of their skin health and improve their overall quality of life.

In the next chapter, we will delve into the role of systemic therapies in the management of folliculitis, including oral antibiotics, oral antifungals, retinoids, and immunomodulators. Understanding the indications, mechanisms of action, and potential side effects of these therapies will further empower readers to make informed decisions about their treatment options and work collaboratively with their healthcare providers to achieve the best possible outcomes.

CHAPTER 9

Chapter 9: Systemic Therapies for Folliculitis

While topical treatments are often the first line of defense against folliculitis, some cases may require the use of systemic therapies to effectively control inflammation, eradicate infectious agents, and prevent recurrent episodes. Systemic therapies, which are medications taken orally or administered through injection or infusion, work by delivering the active ingredients throughout the body, allowing for a more comprehensive approach to treatment. In this chapter, we will explore the various systemic therapies used in the management of folliculitis, including oral antibiotics, oral antifungals, retinoids, and immunomodulators. By understanding the indications, mechanisms of action, and potential side effects of these therapies, individuals with folliculitis can make informed decisions about their treatment options and work collaboratively with their healthcare providers to achieve optimal outcomes.

9.1 Oral Antibiotics

Oral antibiotics are a mainstay of treatment for moderate to severe cases of bacterial folliculitis or those that do not respond to topical therapies alone. These medications work by inhibiting bacterial growth or killing bacteria systemically, helping to clear infections and reduce inflammation.

9.1.1 Types of Oral Antibiotics

Several classes of oral antibiotics are used in the treatment of folliculitis, each with different mechanisms of action and spectrums of activity. Some common oral antibiotics used for folliculitis include:

1. Tetracyclines: Tetracyclines, such as doxycycline and minocycline, are broad-spectrum antibiotics that inhibit bacterial protein synthesis. They are often used as first-line treatments for moderate to severe folliculitis due to their anti-inflammatory properties and effectiveness against a wide range of bacteria, including Staphylococcus aureus.

2. Macrolides: Macrolides, such as erythromycin and azithromycin, also inhibit bacterial protein synthesis and are effective against many gram-positive bacteria. They may be used as alternatives to tetracyclines for individuals who are allergic or unable to tolerate tetracyclines.

3. Beta-lactams: Beta-lactam antibiotics, such as cephalexin and dicloxacillin, work by inhibiting bacterial cell wall synthesis. They are particularly effective against Staphylococcus aureus and may be used for more severe cases of bacterial folliculitis.

4. Fluoroquinolones: Fluoroquinolones, such as ciprofloxacin and levofloxacin, inhibit bacterial DNA gyrase and topoisomerase IV, preventing bacterial replication. They have a broad spectrum of activity and may be used for cases of gram-negative folliculitis or those that do not respond to other antibiotic classes.

9.1.2 Proper Use and Precautions

When using oral antibiotics for folliculitis, it is crucial to follow the prescribed regimen and take necessary precautions to ensure effective treatment and minimize the risk of adverse effects or antibiotic resistance. Some tips for proper use include:

1. Take as directed: Follow the dosage and duration of treatment as prescribed by your healthcare provider. Do not skip doses or stop treatment early, even if symptoms improve, as this can lead to antibiotic resistance or recurrent infections.

2. Take with food: Some oral antibiotics, such as doxycycline, should be taken with food to minimize gastrointestinal side effects. Follow the instructions provided with your medication.

3. Stay hydrated: Drink plenty of water while taking oral antibiotics to prevent dehydration and maintain proper kidney function.

4. Use sun protection: Some antibiotics, particularly tetracyclines, can increase skin sensitivity to sunlight. Use a broad-spectrum sunscreen and protective clothing when taking these medications.

Precautions to keep in mind when using oral antibiotics include:

1. Potential for side effects: Oral antibiotics can cause various side effects, such as gastrointestinal upset, diarrhea, or allergic reactions. Inform your healthcare provider if you experience any concerning symptoms while taking these medications.

2. Drug interactions: Some oral antibiotics may interact with other medications, such as oral contraceptives or blood thinners. Inform your healthcare provider of all medications you are taking before starting treatment with oral antibiotics.

3. Antibiotic resistance: Overuse or misuse of oral antibiotics can contribute to the development of antibiotic-resistant bacteria. Use these medications only as prescribed and for the recommended duration to minimize the risk of resistance.

Regular follow-up with your healthcare provider is essential when using oral antibiotics for folliculitis to monitor treatment response, adjust therapy as needed, and address any concerns or side effects that may arise.

9.2 Oral Antifungals

Oral antifungals are used for the treatment of folliculitis caused by fungal infections, such as Malassezia folliculitis or dermatophyte infections, that are widespread, severe, or resistant to topical therapies. These medications work by inhibiting fungal growth or killing fungi systemically, helping to clear infections and prevent recurrence.

9.2.1 Types of Oral Antifungals

Several classes of oral antifungals are used in the treatment of fungal folliculitis, each with different mechanisms of action and spectrums of activity. Some common oral antifungals used for folliculitis include:

1. Azoles: Azoles, such as itraconazole and fluconazole, inhibit the synthesis of ergosterol, a key component of fungal cell membranes. They are effective against a wide range of fungal species, including Malassezia and dermatophytes, and are often used as first-line treatments for fungal folliculitis.

2. Allylamines: Allylamines, such as terbinafine, inhibit the enzyme squalene epoxidase, disrupting fungal cell membrane synthesis. They have particularly strong activity against dermatophytes and may be used for cases of dermatophyte folliculitis.

3. Griseofulvin: Griseofulvin interferes with fungal cell division by disrupting microtubule formation. It is primarily effective against dermatophytes and may be used for cases of dermatophyte folliculitis that do not respond to other antifungal classes.

9.2.2 Proper Use and Precautions

When using oral antifungals for folliculitis, it is essential to follow the prescribed regimen and take necessary precautions to ensure effective treatment and minimize the risk of adverse effects or treatment failure. Some tips for proper use include:

1. Take as directed: Follow the dosage and duration of treatment as prescribed by your healthcare provider. Some oral antifungals may require a longer course of treatment than others, ranging from several weeks to several months.

2. Take with food: Some oral antifungals, such as itraconazole, should be taken with food to enhance absorption. Follow the instructions provided with your medication.

3. Avoid alcohol: Some oral antifungals, particularly griseofulvin, can cause a disulfiram-like reaction when consumed with alcohol, leading to flushing, nausea, and vomiting. Avoid alcohol while taking these medications.

4. Monitor for side effects: Inform your healthcare provider if you experience any concerning symptoms, such as liver dysfunction, visual disturbances, or skin rash, while taking oral antifungals.

Precautions to keep in mind when using oral antifungals include:

1. Potential for drug interactions: Oral antifungals can interact with various medications, such as blood thinners, immunosuppressants, or certain cardiovascular drugs. Inform your healthcare provider of all medications you are taking before starting treatment with oral antifungals.

2. Liver toxicity: Some oral antifungals, particularly azoles, can cause liver toxicity. Your healthcare provider may monitor your liver function through

blood tests during treatment.

3. Pregnancy and breastfeeding: Some oral antifungals may not be safe for use during pregnancy or breastfeeding. Discuss the risks and benefits of treatment with your healthcare provider if you are pregnant, planning to become pregnant, or breastfeeding.

Regular follow-up with your healthcare provider is crucial when using oral antifungals for folliculitis to monitor treatment response, adjust therapy as needed, and address any concerns or side effects that may arise.

9.3 Retinoids

Retinoids are a class of medications derived from vitamin A that are primarily used for the treatment of acne and other disorders of keratinization. However, they may also be useful in the management of certain types of folliculitis, particularly those associated with follicular occlusion or hyperkeratosis.

9.3.1 Types of Retinoids

Two main types of retinoids are used in the treatment of folliculitis:

1. Isotretinoin: Isotretinoin is an oral retinoid that works by reducing sebum production, normalizing follicular keratinization, and decreasing inflammation. It is typically used for severe, recalcitrant cases of acne but may also be effective for certain types of folliculitis, such as gram-negative folliculitis or folliculitis decalvans.

2. Acitretin: Acitretin is an oral retinoid that is primarily used for the treatment of psoriasis. However, it may also be helpful in managing certain types of folliculitis, particularly those associated with disorders of keratinization, such as pityriasis rubra pilaris or lichen planopilaris.

9.3.2 Proper Use and Precautions

When using retinoids for folliculitis, it is crucial to follow the prescribed regimen and take necessary precautions to ensure effective treatment and minimize the risk of adverse effects. Some tips for proper use include:

1. Take as directed: Follow the dosage and duration of treatment as prescribed by your healthcare provider. Retinoids are typically taken once or twice daily with meals.

2. Use sun protection: Retinoids can increase skin sensitivity to sunlight, leading to an increased risk of sunburn or skin damage. Always use a broad-spectrum sunscreen with an SPF of at least 30 and protective clothing when taking these medications.

3. Avoid pregnancy: Retinoids are teratogenic and can cause severe birth defects. Women of childbearing age must use effective contraception before, during, and after treatment with retinoids. Pregnancy tests may be required before and during treatment.

4. Monitor for side effects: Inform your healthcare provider if you experience any concerning symptoms, such as severe dryness of the skin or mucous membranes, headaches, or visual disturbances, while taking retinoids.

Precautions to keep in mind when using retinoids include:

1. Potential for side effects: Retinoids can cause various side effects, such as dry skin, chapped lips, nosebleeds, or muscle aches. These side effects are usually dose-dependent and may improve with time or dose adjustment.

2. Liver toxicity: Retinoids can cause liver toxicity, particularly at higher doses or in individuals with pre-existing liver disease. Your healthcare provider may monitor your liver function through blood tests during

treatment.

3. Psychiatric effects: In rare cases, retinoids may cause or exacerbate psychiatric symptoms, such as depression or suicidal thoughts. Inform your healthcare provider if you experience any changes in mood or behavior while taking these medications.

Regular follow-up with your healthcare provider is essential when using retinoids for folliculitis to monitor treatment response, adjust therapy as needed, and address any concerns or side effects that may arise.

9.4 Immunomodulators

Immunomodulators are medications that modify the immune system's response and are used in the treatment of various inflammatory and autoimmune disorders. In the context of folliculitis, immunomodulators may be helpful for managing certain types of the condition, particularly those associated with an overactive or dysregulated immune response.

9.4.1 Types of Immunomodulators

Several types of immunomodulators may be used in the treatment of folliculitis, depending on the underlying cause and severity of the condition. Some examples include:

1. Corticosteroids: Oral corticosteroids, such as prednisone, work by suppressing inflammation and modulating the immune response. They may be used for short courses to control acute flares of severe or widespread folliculitis, particularly in cases of eosinophilic folliculitis or folliculitis decalvans.

2. Dapsone: Dapsone is an antimicrobial and anti-inflammatory medication that is often used for the treatment of dermatitis herpetiformis and other

inflammatory skin disorders. It may also be effective for certain types of folliculitis, such as eosinophilic folliculitis or folliculitis in individuals with HIV/AIDS.

3. Cyclosporine: Cyclosporine is an immunosuppressant medication that inhibits T-cell activation and cytokine production. It may be used for severe or recalcitrant cases of folliculitis, particularly those associated with underlying inflammatory or autoimmune disorders.

4. Biologics: Biologic agents, such as adalimumab or infliximab, are targeted immunomodulators that inhibit specific cytokines or immune pathways. They may be used for severe or treatment-resistant cases of folliculitis associated with conditions like hidradenitis suppurativa or Crohn's disease.

9.4.2 Proper Use and Precautions

When using immunomodulators for folliculitis, it is essential to follow the prescribed regimen and take necessary precautions to ensure effective treatment and minimize the risk of adverse effects. Some tips for proper use include:

1. Take as directed: Follow the dosage and duration of treatment as prescribed by your healthcare provider. Some immunomodulators may require regular blood tests to monitor for potential side effects or adjust dosage.

2. Be aware of infection risks: Immunomodulators can increase the risk of infections, including serious or opportunistic infections. Report any signs of infection, such as fever, chills, or persistent cough, to your healthcare provider promptly.

3. Use sun protection: Some immunomodulators, particularly cyclosporine, can increase skin sensitivity to sunlight. Use a broad-spectrum sunscreen and protective clothing when taking these medications.

4. Inform your healthcare provider of other medications: Immunomodulators can interact with various medications, such as antibiotics, antifungals, or blood pressure medications. Inform your healthcare provider of all medications you are taking before starting treatment with immunomodulators.

Precautions to keep in mind when using immunomodulators include:

1. Potential for side effects: Immunomodulators can cause various side effects, such as gastrointestinal upset, headaches, or tremors. These side effects may vary depending on the specific medication and dosage used.

2. Long-term risks: Some immunomodulators, particularly cyclosporine, may be associated with an increased risk of certain cancers or kidney toxicity with long-term use. Your healthcare provider will weigh the benefits and risks of treatment and monitor you closely for any potential complications.

3. Pregnancy and breastfeeding: Some immunomodulators may not be safe for use during pregnancy or breastfeeding. Discuss the risks and benefits of treatment with your healthcare provider if you are pregnant, planning to become pregnant, or breastfeeding.

Regular follow-up with your healthcare provider is crucial when using immunomodulators for folliculitis to monitor treatment response, adjust therapy as needed, and address any concerns or side effects that may arise.

Conclusion

Systemic therapies play a critical role in the management of moderate to severe cases of folliculitis or those that do not respond to topical treatments alone. Oral antibiotics, oral antifungals, retinoids, and immunomodulators each offer unique mechanisms of action and potential benefits for individuals with folliculitis, depending on the underlying cause and severity of the condition.

When considering systemic therapies for folliculitis, it is essential to work closely with a healthcare provider to carefully weigh the potential benefits and risks of treatment. Factors such as the type and extent of folliculitis, individual medical history, and potential for side effects or drug interactions should be taken into account when developing a personalized treatment plan.

Proper use of systemic therapies, including adhering to prescribed regimens, monitoring for side effects, and attending regular follow-up appointments, is crucial for ensuring effective treatment and minimizing the risk of adverse outcomes. By staying informed and actively engaged in their care, individuals with folliculitis can work collaboratively with their healthcare providers to achieve optimal skin health and quality of life.

As we continue to explore the various treatment options for folliculitis, it is important to remember that a comprehensive approach, incorporating both topical and systemic therapies, lifestyle modifications, and patient education, is often necessary for successful long-term management. By staying up-to-date on the latest research and treatment advances, healthcare providers and individuals with folliculitis can work together to develop innovative and effective strategies for managing this challenging condition.

In the next chapter, we will delve into the role of light and laser therapies in the treatment of folliculitis, including photodynamic therapy, pulsed dye laser, Nd:YAG laser, and intense pulsed light. Understanding the mechanisms of action, potential benefits, and limitations of these therapies will provide readers with a more comprehensive understanding of the full range of treatment options available for folliculitis.

CHAPTER 10

Chapter 10: Light and Laser Therapies

As our understanding of the pathogenesis and management of folliculitis continues to evolve, light and laser therapies have emerged as promising treatment options for certain types of the condition. These therapies offer a targeted, non-invasive approach to reducing inflammation, eliminating infectious agents, and improving the overall appearance of the skin. In this chapter, we will explore the various light and laser therapies used in the treatment of folliculitis, including photodynamic therapy (PDT), pulsed dye laser (PDL), neodymium-doped yttrium aluminum garnet (Nd:YAG) laser, and intense pulsed light (IPL). By understanding the mechanisms of action, potential benefits, and limitations of these therapies, healthcare providers and individuals with folliculitis can make informed decisions about incorporating light and laser treatments into their comprehensive management plans.

10.1 Photodynamic Therapy

Photodynamic therapy (PDT) is a two-step treatment that combines the use of a photosensitizing agent with exposure to a specific wavelength of light to selectively target and destroy abnormal cells while sparing healthy tissue. In the context of folliculitis, PDT may be particularly useful for treating cases associated with bacterial or fungal infections, as well as those with follicular occlusion or hyperkeratosis.

10.1.1 Mechanism of Action

The PDT process involves the following steps:

1. Application of a photosensitizing agent: A photosensitizing agent, such as aminolevulinic acid (ALA) or methyl aminolevulinate (MAL), is applied to the affected skin and allowed to incubate for a specific period, typically ranging from 30 minutes to several hours. During this time, the photosensitizer is preferentially absorbed by rapidly dividing cells, such as those in hair follicles or inflammatory lesions.

2. Exposure to light: The treated area is then exposed to a specific wavelength of light, usually in the blue or red spectrum, which activates the photosensitizer. This activation leads to the production of reactive oxygen species, which cause localized damage to the targeted cells, leading to their destruction.

3. Healing and recovery: Following PDT, the treated area may experience some redness, swelling, and peeling as the damaged cells are replaced by healthy tissue. This process typically takes several days to a week, and the skin may be more sensitive to sunlight during this time.

10.1.2 Indications and Efficacy

PDT may be considered for the treatment of folliculitis in the following situations:

1. Bacterial folliculitis: PDT has been shown to be effective in reducing the bacterial load and improving the appearance of the skin in cases of recurrent or treatment-resistant bacterial folliculitis, particularly those caused by Staphylococcus aureus or Propionibacterium acnes.

2. Fungal folliculitis: PDT may also be useful for treating fungal folliculitis,

such as Malassezia folliculitis, by targeting the fungal elements within the hair follicles and reducing inflammation.

3. Follicular occlusion: In cases of folliculitis associated with follicular occlusion or hyperkeratosis, such as folliculitis decalvans or lichen planopilaris, PDT may help to improve the penetration of topical medications and promote the normalization of follicular keratinization.

The efficacy of PDT for folliculitis has been demonstrated in several studies, with improvements in clinical symptoms, quality of life, and long-term remission rates. However, the response to treatment may vary depending on the type and severity of folliculitis, as well as individual patient factors.

10.1.3 Advantages and Limitations

Some advantages of PDT for the treatment of folliculitis include:

1. Targeted therapy: PDT allows for the selective targeting of abnormal cells within the hair follicles, minimizing damage to surrounding healthy tissue.

2. Minimal systemic side effects: Unlike oral medications, PDT has limited systemic absorption and fewer potential side effects.

3. Combination with other therapies: PDT can be used in combination with other topical or systemic therapies to enhance treatment outcomes.

However, there are also some limitations to consider:

1. Discomfort during treatment: The activation of the photosensitizer can cause a burning or stinging sensation, which may be uncomfortable for some patients.

2. Downtime after treatment: The treated area may be red, swollen, and

peeling for several days after PDT, which may require some social downtime.

3. Need for multiple treatments: Depending on the type and severity of folliculitis, multiple PDT sessions may be necessary to achieve optimal results.

10.2 Pulsed Dye Laser

Pulsed dye laser (PDL) is a type of vascular laser that targets hemoglobin within blood vessels, leading to the selective destruction of abnormal vasculature while preserving the surrounding tissue. In the context of folliculitis, PDL may be particularly useful for treating cases associated with inflammation, erythema, or scarring.

10.2.1 Mechanism of Action

PDL emits a specific wavelength of light, typically in the yellow spectrum (585-595 nm), which is preferentially absorbed by hemoglobin within the blood vessels. As the laser energy is absorbed, it causes localized heating and damage to the blood vessels, leading to their coagulation and collapse. This process can help to reduce inflammation, improve the appearance of erythema, and promote the remodeling of scar tissue.

10.2.2 Indications and Efficacy

PDL may be considered for the treatment of folliculitis in the following situations:

1. Inflammatory folliculitis: In cases of folliculitis associated with significant inflammation and erythema, such as eosinophilic folliculitis or folliculitis keloidalis nuchae, PDL can help to reduce the vascular component and improve the overall appearance of the skin.

2. Scarring folliculitis: PDL may also be useful for treating cases of folliculitis

that have resulted in scarring, such as folliculitis decalvans or dissecting cellulitis of the scalp. By targeting the abnormal blood vessels within the scars, PDL can help to soften and flatten the scar tissue over time.

Several studies have demonstrated the efficacy of PDL for improving the clinical symptoms and appearance of folliculitis, with some patients achieving long-term remission. However, the response to treatment may vary depending on the type and severity of folliculitis, as well as individual patient factors.

10.2.3 Advantages and Limitations

Some advantages of PDL for the treatment of folliculitis include:

1. Non-invasive therapy: PDL is a non-invasive treatment that does not require any incisions or injections, making it a well-tolerated option for many patients.

2. Minimal downtime: Most patients experience only mild redness and swelling after PDL treatment, which typically resolves within a few days.

3. Combination with other therapies: PDL can be used in combination with other topical or systemic therapies to enhance treatment outcomes.

However, there are also some limitations to consider:

1. Discomfort during treatment: Some patients may experience a snapping or burning sensation during PDL treatment, although this can be minimized with the use of cooling devices or topical anesthetics.

2. Need for multiple treatments: Depending on the type and severity of folliculitis, multiple PDL sessions may be necessary to achieve optimal results.

3. Potential for pigmentary changes: In some cases, particularly in patients with darker skin types, PDL may cause temporary or permanent changes in skin pigmentation.

10.3 Nd:YAG Laser

Neodymium-doped yttrium aluminum garnet (Nd:YAG) laser is a type of laser that can penetrate deeper into the skin compared to other laser types, making it useful for targeting structures within the dermis, such as hair follicles and inflammatory lesions. In the context of folliculitis, Nd:YAG laser may be particularly useful for treating cases associated with deep inflammation or hair follicle destruction.

10.3.1 Mechanism of Action

Nd:YAG laser emits a specific wavelength of light, typically in the near-infrared spectrum (1064 nm), which can penetrate deeper into the skin compared to other laser wavelengths. As the laser energy is absorbed by the target structures, such as hair follicles or inflammatory cells, it causes localized heating and damage, leading to their destruction. This process can help to reduce inflammation, decrease the bacterial load within the hair follicles, and promote the healing of damaged tissue.

10.3.2 Indications and Efficacy

Nd:YAG laser may be considered for the treatment of folliculitis in the following situations:

1. Deep folliculitis: In cases of folliculitis involving the deeper portions of the hair follicles, such as sycosis barbae or folliculitis decalvans, Nd:YAG laser can help to target the inflammatory cells and reduce the severity of the condition.

2. Gram-negative folliculitis: Nd:YAG laser may also be useful for treating cases of gram-negative folliculitis, which can be resistant to conventional antibiotic therapy. By reducing the bacterial load within the hair follicles, Nd:YAG laser can help to improve the clinical symptoms and prevent recurrences.

3. Pseudofolliculitis barbae: In cases of pseudofolliculitis barbae, or "razor bumps," Nd:YAG laser can be used to destroy the hair follicles and prevent the regrowth of curved hairs that can cause inflammation and bumps.

Several studies have demonstrated the efficacy of Nd:YAG laser for improving the clinical symptoms and appearance of various types of folliculitis, with some patients achieving long-term remission. However, the response to treatment may vary depending on the type and severity of folliculitis, as well as individual patient factors.

10.3.3 Advantages and Limitations

Some advantages of Nd:YAG laser for the treatment of folliculitis include:

1. Deep tissue penetration: The longer wavelength of Nd:YAG laser allows for deeper penetration into the skin, making it useful for targeting structures within the dermis.

2. Versatility: Nd:YAG laser can be used to treat a variety of folliculitis types, as well as other inflammatory skin conditions.

3. Combination with other therapies: Nd:YAG laser can be used in combination with other topical or systemic therapies to enhance treatment outcomes.

However, there are also some limitations to consider:

1. Discomfort during treatment: Some patients may experience a burning or stinging sensation during Nd:YAG laser treatment, although this can be minimized with the use of cooling devices or topical anesthetics.

2. Need for multiple treatments: Depending on the type and severity of folliculitis, multiple Nd:YAG laser sessions may be necessary to achieve optimal results.

3. Potential for pigmentary changes: In some cases, particularly in patients with darker skin types, Nd:YAG laser may cause temporary or permanent changes in skin pigmentation.

10.4 Intense Pulsed Light (IPL)

Intense pulsed light (IPL) is a type of broadband light therapy that emits multiple wavelengths of light, allowing for the targeting of various structures within the skin, such as blood vessels, pigment, and hair follicles. In the context of folliculitis, IPL may be particularly useful for treating cases associated with inflammation, erythema, or hyperpigmentation.

10.4.1 Mechanism of Action

IPL devices emit a broad spectrum of light, typically in the visible and near-infrared range (400-1200 nm). By using filters, the wavelengths of light can be customized to target specific structures within the skin. As the light energy is absorbed by the target structures, such as hemoglobin in blood vessels or melanin in pigmented lesions, it causes localized heating and damage, leading to their destruction or remodeling. This process can help to reduce inflammation, improve the appearance of erythema and hyperpigmentation, and promote the healing of damaged tissue.

10.4.2 Indications and Efficacy

IPL may be considered for the treatment of folliculitis in the following situations:

1. Inflammatory folliculitis: In cases of folliculitis associated with significant inflammation and erythema, such as eosinophilic folliculitis or folliculitis keloidalis nuchae, IPL can help to reduce the vascular component and improve the overall appearance of the skin.

2. Post-inflammatory hyperpigmentation: IPL may also be useful for treating cases of folliculitis that have resulted in post-inflammatory hyperpigmentation, as the light energy can target the excess melanin and help to even out the skin tone.

3. Recurrent folliculitis: By targeting the hair follicles and reducing the bacterial load, IPL may help to prevent the recurrence of certain types of folliculitis, such as pseudofolliculitis barbae or folliculitis decalvans.

Several studies have demonstrated the efficacy of IPL for improving the clinical symptoms and appearance of various types of folliculitis, with some patients achieving long-term remission. However, the response to treatment may vary depending on the type and severity of folliculitis, as well as individual patient factors.

10.4.3 Advantages and Limitations

Some advantages of IPL for the treatment of folliculitis include:

1. Versatility: IPL can be customized to target various structures within the skin, making it useful for treating a variety of folliculitis types and associated conditions, such as erythema or hyperpigmentation.

2. Larger treatment areas: IPL devices can treat larger areas of the skin compared to some laser types, making it more efficient for treating extensive

or multiple folliculitis lesions.

3. Combination with other therapies: IPL can be used in combination with other topical or systemic therapies to enhance treatment outcomes.

However, there are also some limitations to consider:

1. Discomfort during treatment: Some patients may experience a burning or stinging sensation during IPL treatment, although this can be minimized with the use of cooling devices or topical anesthetics.

2. Need for multiple treatments: Depending on the type and severity of folliculitis, multiple IPL sessions may be necessary to achieve optimal results.

3. Potential for pigmentary changes: In some cases, particularly in patients with darker skin types, IPL may cause temporary or permanent changes in skin pigmentation, although this risk can be minimized with proper patient selection and device settings.

Conclusion

Light and laser therapies offer a promising approach to the treatment of various types of folliculitis, providing targeted therapy with minimal systemic side effects. Photodynamic therapy, pulsed dye laser, Nd:YAG laser, and intense pulsed light each have unique mechanisms of action and potential benefits for patients with folliculitis, depending on the specific type and severity of the condition.

When considering light and laser therapies for folliculitis, healthcare providers should carefully evaluate the individual patient's presentation, medical history, and treatment goals to determine the most appropriate modality. Factors such as skin type, lesion depth and extent, and potential for adverse effects should be taken into account when developing a personalized treatment plan.

Patients undergoing light and laser therapies for folliculitis should be counseled on the expected treatment course, potential side effects, and necessary precautions, such as sun protection and skin care. Regular follow-up with the treating provider is essential to monitor treatment response, adjust therapy as needed, and address any concerns that may arise.

As research into the use of light and laser therapies for folliculitis continues to evolve, it is crucial for healthcare providers to stay up-to-date on the latest evidence and best practices. By incorporating these advanced treatment modalities into a comprehensive management plan, providers can offer patients with folliculitis new hope for achieving clear, healthy skin and improved quality of life.

Looking ahead, the next chapter will explore the critical role of prevention strategies in the management of folliculitis. From skin hygiene and cleansing to hair removal techniques and lifestyle modifications, we will discuss the evidence-based approaches that can help patients reduce their risk of developing or exacerbating folliculitis. By empowering patients with the knowledge and tools to take proactive steps in their skin health, we can work towards a future where folliculitis is not only effectively treated but also successfully prevented.

CHAPTER 11

C hapter 11: Prevention Strategies for Folliculitis

While effective treatment options are essential for managing folliculitis, preventing the development or recurrence of the condition is equally crucial. By adopting evidence-based prevention strategies, individuals can take proactive steps to maintain healthy skin and minimize the risk of folliculitis outbreaks. In this chapter, we will explore the key pillars of folliculitis prevention, including skin hygiene and cleansing, hair removal techniques, clothing and fabric choices, and lifestyle modifications. By incorporating these strategies into their daily routines, patients can work towards achieving long-term control of folliculitis and improving their overall skin health.

11.1 Skin Hygiene and Cleansing

Proper skin hygiene and cleansing are the foundation of folliculitis prevention. By keeping the skin clean and free of excess oils, sweat, and bacteria, individuals can reduce the likelihood of hair follicles becoming clogged or infected. However, it is essential to strike a balance between effective cleansing and maintaining the skin's natural protective barrier.

11.1.1 Gentle Cleansing

When cleansing the skin, it is important to use gentle, non-irritating products that do not disrupt the skin's natural pH or strip away beneficial oils. Some tips for gentle cleansing include:

1. Using lukewarm water: Hot water can be drying and irritating to the skin, so it is best to use lukewarm water when cleansing.

2. Choosing mild, fragrance-free cleansers: Look for cleansers that are specifically designed for sensitive skin and do not contain harsh surfactants, alcohol, or fragrances.

3. Avoiding excessive scrubbing: Rubbing the skin too vigorously can cause irritation and damage to the hair follicles. Instead, use gentle, circular motions when cleansing.

4. Patting dry: After cleansing, gently pat the skin dry with a clean, soft towel rather than rubbing, which can cause friction and irritation.

11.1.2 Moisturizing

Keeping the skin properly hydrated is essential for maintaining its barrier function and preventing folliculitis. After cleansing, individuals should apply a non-comedogenic, fragrance-free moisturizer to help lock in hydration and protect the skin from external irritants. Those with particularly dry or sensitive skin may benefit from using a thicker, cream-based moisturizer, while those with oily or acne-prone skin may prefer a lighter, gel-based formula.

11.1.3 Antimicrobial Cleansers

For individuals with recurrent or difficult-to-control folliculitis, using antimicrobial cleansers containing ingredients such as benzoyl peroxide, salicylic acid, or chlorhexidine may be beneficial. These ingredients can help to reduce the bacterial load on the skin and prevent the development of new folliculitis lesions. However, it is important to use these products as directed and not to overuse them, as they can be drying or irritating to the skin if used too frequently or in too high concentrations.

11.1.4 Exfoliation

Regular exfoliation can help to remove dead skin cells and prevent the buildup of excess keratin around the hair follicles, which can contribute to folliculitis. However, it is important to choose gentle exfoliation methods and not to overdo it, as excessive exfoliation can cause irritation and damage to the skin. Some gentle exfoliation options include:

1. Using a soft-bristled brush or loofah: Gently brushing the skin in circular motions can help to remove dead skin cells and improve circulation.

2. Applying a chemical exfoliant: Products containing alpha-hydroxy acids (AHAs) or beta-hydroxy acids (BHAs) can help to dissolve dead skin cells and unclog hair follicles. However, these products should be used sparingly and as directed, as they can be irritating to sensitive skin.

3. Trying a mild physical exfoliant: Scrubs containing fine, gentle particles such as jojoba beads or rice powder can help to physically remove dead skin cells without causing excessive abrasion.

11.2 Hair Removal Techniques

Hair removal is a common trigger for folliculitis, particularly in areas where the hair is coarse or curly, such as the beard area, pubic region, or legs. By adopting proper hair removal techniques and taking steps to minimize irritation, individuals can reduce their risk of developing folliculitis.

11.2.1 Shaving

Shaving is one of the most common hair removal methods and can be a major trigger for folliculitis, particularly in individuals with curly or coarse hair. To minimize the risk of folliculitis when shaving, consider the following tips:

1. Using a sharp, clean razor: Dull or dirty razors can cause more irritation and increase the risk of infection. Be sure to use a sharp, clean razor and replace the blade frequently.

2. Applying shaving cream or gel: Using a lubricating shaving cream or gel can help the razor glide more smoothly over the skin and reduce friction and irritation.

3. Shaving in the direction of hair growth: Shaving against the grain can cause the hair to be cut too closely, increasing the risk of ingrown hairs and folliculitis.

4. Rinsing the blade after each stroke: Rinsing the razor blade with warm water after each stroke can help to remove shaving cream, hair, and bacteria that can contribute to folliculitis.

5. Applying a cool compress: After shaving, applying a cool compress to the area can help to soothe the skin and reduce inflammation.

11.2.2 Waxing and Plucking

Waxing and plucking are hair removal methods that involve pulling the hair out by the root. While these methods can provide longer-lasting results than shaving, they can also be more irritating to the skin and increase the risk of folliculitis. To minimize the risk of folliculitis when waxing or plucking, consider the following tips:

1. Ensuring proper hygiene: Be sure to use clean, disposable applicators and wax that has not been double-dipped to avoid the spread of bacteria.

2. Applying a pre-wax cleanser: Using a pre-wax cleanser can help to remove excess oils and bacteria from the skin, reducing the risk of infection.

3. Avoiding hot wax: Wax that is too hot can burn the skin and increase inflammation. Be sure to test the temperature of the wax before applying it to the skin.

4. Applying a soothing post-wax product: After waxing or plucking, applying a soothing, antiseptic product containing ingredients such as aloe vera or tea tree oil can help to calm the skin and prevent infection.

11.2.3 Laser Hair Removal

Laser hair removal is a long-term hair reduction method that uses targeted laser energy to destroy the hair follicles. While laser hair removal can be an effective way to reduce the frequency of hair removal and minimize the risk of folliculitis, it is important to choose a reputable provider and follow proper pre- and post-treatment guidelines. Some tips for minimizing the risk of folliculitis with laser hair removal include:

1. Avoiding sun exposure: It is important to avoid sun exposure and tanning for at least four weeks before and after laser hair removal, as this can increase the risk of skin irritation and folliculitis.

2. Following pre-treatment instructions: Before laser hair removal, patients should avoid waxing, plucking, or threading the treatment area and should shave the hair down to a stubble to allow the laser to target the follicles.

3. Using a cool compress: After laser hair removal, applying a cool compress to the treated area can help to reduce inflammation and minimize the risk of folliculitis.

4. Avoiding tight clothing: Wearing loose, breathable clothing after laser hair

removal can help to reduce friction and irritation on the treated area.

11.3 Clothing and Fabric Choices

The clothing and fabrics that come into contact with the skin can play a significant role in the development or exacerbation of folliculitis. By making strategic clothing and fabric choices, individuals can help to minimize friction, irritation, and the buildup of sweat and bacteria that can contribute to folliculitis.

11.3.1 Breathable Fabrics

Choosing clothing made from breathable, moisture-wicking fabrics can help to keep the skin dry and reduce the risk of folliculitis. Some examples of breathable fabrics include:

1. Cotton: Cotton is a natural, lightweight fabric that allows air to circulate and moisture to evaporate, making it a good choice for individuals with folliculitis.

2. Bamboo: Bamboo fabric is naturally antibacterial and moisture-wicking, making it a good choice for activewear or clothing worn close to the skin.

3. Merino wool: Merino wool is a lightweight, breathable fabric that can help to regulate body temperature and reduce the buildup of sweat and bacteria.

11.3.2 Loose-Fitting Clothing

Wearing loose-fitting clothing can help to reduce friction and irritation on the skin, which can contribute to the development of folliculitis. Tight clothing, particularly in areas where the skin rubs together such as the thighs or underarms, can trap sweat and bacteria and increase the risk of infection. When choosing clothing, look for styles that allow the skin to breathe and do not fit too snugly against the body.

11.3.3 Avoiding Irritating Fabrics

Certain fabrics and clothing materials can be irritating to the skin and increase the risk of folliculitis. Some examples of potentially irritating fabrics include:

1. Wool: While merino wool is generally well-tolerated, other types of wool can be rough and scratchy, causing irritation and inflammation of the hair follicles.

2. Synthetic fabrics: Some synthetic fabrics, such as polyester or nylon, can trap sweat and bacteria against the skin and cause irritation, particularly in individuals with sensitive skin.

3. Rough or abrasive materials: Clothing with rough seams, tags, or embellishments can rub against the skin and cause irritation, increasing the risk of folliculitis.

11.3.4 Changing Out of Sweaty Clothing

After exercising or sweating heavily, it is important to change out of damp clothing as soon as possible to reduce the risk of folliculitis. Sweaty clothing can trap moisture and bacteria against the skin, creating an ideal environment for the development of infection. By changing into clean, dry clothing and showering promptly after sweating, individuals can help to minimize the risk of folliculitis.

11.4 Lifestyle Modifications

In addition to skin hygiene, hair removal, and clothing choices, certain lifestyle modifications can also play a role in preventing folliculitis. By making strategic changes to diet, exercise, and other daily habits, individuals can help to support skin health and reduce the risk of folliculitis outbreaks.

11.4.1 Diet and Nutrition

While there is no specific diet that has been proven to prevent folliculitis, eating a balanced, nutrient-rich diet can help to support overall skin health and immune function. Some dietary tips for preventing folliculitis include:

1. Staying hydrated: Drinking plenty of water and other hydrating fluids can help to keep the skin moisturized and flush out toxins that can contribute to inflammation.

2. Eating a rainbow of fruits and vegetables: Colorful fruits and vegetables are rich in antioxidants and other nutrients that can help to support skin health and reduce inflammation.

3. Choosing healthy fats: Healthy fats, such as those found in fatty fish, nuts, and seeds, can help to nourish the skin and reduce inflammation.

4. Limiting sugar and processed foods: Consuming a diet high in sugar and processed foods can contribute to inflammation and may exacerbate folliculitis in some individuals.

11.4.2 Exercise and Sweat Management

Regular exercise is important for overall health and can also help to improve circulation and support skin health. However, sweating during exercise can also increase the risk of folliculitis if proper hygiene measures are not taken. To minimize the risk of folliculitis during exercise, consider the following tips:

1. Wearing moisture-wicking clothing: Choosing exercise clothing made

from breathable, moisture-wicking fabrics can help to keep sweat away from the skin and reduce the risk of irritation and infection.

2. Showering promptly after exercise: Showering as soon as possible after exercising can help to remove sweat, bacteria, and other debris from the skin and hair follicles.

3. Using a clean towel: Be sure to use a clean towel to dry off after showering and avoid sharing towels with others, as this can spread bacteria and increase the risk of infection.

4. Disinfecting shared equipment: If using shared exercise equipment, such as yoga mats or weight benches, be sure to disinfect the surface before and after use to minimize the spread of bacteria.

11.4.3 Stress Management

Chronic stress can take a toll on the skin and may exacerbate folliculitis in some individuals. When the body is under stress, it produces hormones such as cortisol that can increase inflammation and suppress immune function, making the skin more vulnerable to infection. To minimize the impact of stress on folliculitis, consider the following stress management techniques:

1. Practicing relaxation techniques: Techniques such as deep breathing, meditation, or yoga can help to reduce stress and promote relaxation.

2. Getting enough sleep: Aim to get 7-9 hours of quality sleep each night to support immune function and overall health.

3. Engaging in hobbies and activities: Participating in enjoyable hobbies and activities can help to reduce stress and promote a sense of well-being.

4. Seeking support: Talking to friends, family members, or a mental health

professional can help to manage stress and provide a sense of support and connection.

11.4.4 Avoiding Triggers

For some individuals, certain triggers such as heat, humidity, or friction can exacerbate folliculitis. By identifying and avoiding these triggers, individuals can help to minimize the risk of outbreaks. Some common triggers to consider include:

1. Hot tubs and swimming pools: Poorly maintained hot tubs and swimming pools can harbor bacteria that can cause folliculitis. If using these facilities, be sure to shower immediately after and avoid sitting in wet clothing.

2. Tight clothing: Wearing tight clothing, particularly in areas where the skin rubs together, can increase friction and irritation and contribute to the development of folliculitis.

3. Harsh skincare products: Using skincare products that are too harsh or irritating can disrupt the skin's natural barrier and increase the risk of infection. Choose gentle, non-comedogenic products that are appropriate for your skin type.

4. Certain medications: Some medications, such as corticosteroids or immunosuppressants, can increase the risk of folliculitis. If you are taking these medications and experiencing frequent outbreaks, talk to your healthcare provider about potential alternatives or preventive measures.

Conclusion

Preventing folliculitis requires a multi-faceted approach that incorporates skin hygiene, hair removal techniques, clothing and fabric choices, and lifestyle modifications. By taking a proactive approach to skin health and making strategic changes to daily routines, individuals can help to minimize the risk of folliculitis outbreaks and maintain healthy, clear skin.

Some key takeaways from this chapter include:

1. Proper skin hygiene, including gentle cleansing, moisturizing, and targeted use of antimicrobial products, can help to reduce the risk of folliculitis.

2. Adopting appropriate hair removal techniques, such as using sharp, clean razors and avoiding excessive waxing or plucking, can minimize irritation and inflammation of the hair follicles.

3. Choosing breathable, non-irritating clothing and fabrics and changing out of sweaty clothing promptly can help to reduce friction and the buildup of sweat and bacteria on the skin.

4. Making lifestyle modifications, such as eating a balanced diet, exercising regularly, managing stress, and avoiding triggers, can support overall skin health and reduce the risk of folliculitis outbreaks.

It is important to remember that prevention strategies may need to be tailored to the individual, taking into account factors such as skin type, medical history, and personal preferences. By working closely with a healthcare provider and staying attuned to the unique needs of their skin, individuals can develop a personalized prevention plan that works for them.

As we move forward in our understanding of folliculitis and its management, ongoing research into prevention strategies will be crucial. By staying up-to-date on the latest evidence and recommendations, healthcare providers can continue to empower patients with the knowledge and tools they need to take control of their skin health and minimize the impact of folliculitis on their daily lives.

Looking ahead, the next chapter will explore the significant impact that folliculitis can have on quality of life, including its psychological and social implications. By understanding the far-reaching effects of this condition, we can work towards developing a more holistic and compassionate approach to folliculitis management that prioritizes not only physical health but also emotional well-being and social support.

CHAPTER 12

C hapter 12: Folliculitis and Quality of Life

Folliculitis, like many chronic skin conditions, can have a profound impact on an individual's quality of life. Beyond the physical symptoms of itching, pain, and discomfort, folliculitis can also take a significant toll on mental health, self-esteem, and social functioning. In this chapter, we will explore the multifaceted ways in which folliculitis can affect quality of life, including its psychological impact, the social stigma and isolation that can accompany the condition, and the challenges of coping with a chronic skin disorder. By understanding the far-reaching effects of folliculitis, healthcare providers and patients alike can work towards developing a more comprehensive and compassionate approach to management that addresses not only the physical aspects of the condition but also its emotional and social implications.

12.1 Psychological Impact of Folliculitis

The psychological impact of folliculitis can be significant and far-reaching, affecting individuals of all ages and backgrounds. From the frustration and disappointment of recurrent outbreaks to the anxiety and self-consciousness that can accompany visible skin lesions, folliculitis can take a heavy emotional toll.

12.1.1 Frustration and Disappointment

For many individuals with folliculitis, the chronic and recurrent nature of the condition can be a significant source of frustration and disappointment. Despite adherence to treatment regimens and preventive measures, flare-ups may still occur, leading to feelings of helplessness and a sense of lack of control over one's own body. This frustration can be compounded by the time and energy required to manage the condition, including frequent doctor's appointments, application of topical treatments, and lifestyle modifications.

12.1.2 Anxiety and Self-Consciousness

Folliculitis lesions, particularly when they occur in visible areas such as the face, neck, or arms, can be a source of significant anxiety and self-consciousness. Individuals may worry about the appearance of their skin and how it will be perceived by others, leading to feelings of embarrassment or shame. This anxiety can be particularly acute in social or professional settings, where individuals may feel the need to hide or cover up their skin.

12.1.3 Depression and Low Self-Esteem

The chronic nature of folliculitis, combined with its impact on appearance and social functioning, can contribute to the development of depression and low self-esteem in some individuals. The persistent discomfort and visible signs of the condition can erode self-confidence and lead to negative self-image, particularly in adolescents and young adults who may already be struggling with issues of identity and self-worth.

12.1.4 Body Image Concerns

Folliculitis can also have a significant impact on body image, particularly when it affects areas of the body that are commonly associated with attractiveness or sexuality, such as the chest, back, or buttocks. Individuals may feel self-conscious about the appearance of their skin in intimate settings or may avoid certain activities, such as swimming or exercise, due to concerns about exposing affected areas.

12.1.5 Addressing Psychological Impact

Given the significant psychological impact that folliculitis can have, it is crucial for healthcare providers to assess and address the emotional well-being of their patients as part of a comprehensive treatment approach. This may involve:

1. Providing education and reassurance: Helping patients understand the nature of their condition and the available treatment options can help to reduce anxiety and promote a sense of control.

2. Screening for mental health concerns: Routinely screening patients with folliculitis for symptoms of depression, anxiety, or other mental health concerns can help to identify individuals who may benefit from additional support or referral to mental health professionals.

3. Encouraging self-care and stress management: Promoting healthy coping strategies, such as stress reduction techniques, regular exercise, and engaging in enjoyable activities, can help to improve overall well-being and resilience.

4. Offering support and resources: Providing patients with information about support groups, online resources, or other forms of social support can help to reduce feelings of isolation and promote a sense of community.

By acknowledging and addressing the psychological impact of folliculitis, healthcare providers can help to improve the overall quality of life for their patients and promote a more holistic approach to management.

12.2 Social Stigma and Self-Esteem

In addition to its psychological impact, folliculitis can also have significant social consequences, particularly when it results in visible skin lesions or scarring. The social stigma associated with skin disorders can lead to feelings of shame, embarrassment, and isolation, further compounding the negative impact of the condition on self-esteem and quality of life.

12.2.1 Stigmatization and Misconceptions

Despite advances in public understanding of skin disorders, there remains a significant amount of stigma and misconception surrounding conditions like folliculitis. Individuals with visible skin lesions may be perceived as unclean, contagious, or unhealthy, leading to negative judgments and discrimination in social or professional settings. This stigmatization can be particularly challenging for adolescents and young adults, who may already be struggling with issues of identity and social acceptance.

12.2.2 Impact on Social Functioning

The social stigma associated with folliculitis can have a significant impact on an individual's social functioning and relationships. Individuals may feel self-conscious or embarrassed about their appearance, leading to avoidance of social situations or activities that involve exposing affected areas of the body. This can lead to feelings of isolation and loneliness, as well as difficulties forming or maintaining friendships or romantic relationships.

12.2.3 Occupational and Educational Challenges

Folliculitis can also pose challenges in occupational and educational settings, particularly when it affects visible areas of the body or results in frequent absences due to flare-ups or treatment appointments. Individuals may face discrimination or negative perceptions from colleagues or supervisors, leading to difficulties with job performance or advancement. Students with folliculitis may struggle with absenteeism or face bullying or teasing from peers, further impacting their academic and social development.

12.2.4 Addressing Social Stigma and Self-Esteem

Addressing the social stigma and self-esteem issues associated with folliculitis requires a multi-faceted approach that involves education, support, and advocacy. Some strategies for addressing these challenges include:

1. Public education and awareness: Promoting greater public understanding of skin disorders like folliculitis can help to reduce stigma and misconceptions. This may involve educational campaigns, media outreach, or partnerships with patient advocacy organizations.

2. Encouraging self-advocacy: Empowering individuals with folliculitis to advocate for themselves and their needs can help to promote greater understanding and acceptance in social and professional settings. This may involve providing training in communication skills, assertiveness, or disability rights.

3. Promoting body positivity: Encouraging individuals with folliculitis to embrace their bodies and celebrate their unique qualities can help to improve self-esteem and reduce the impact of social stigma. This may involve promoting positive self-talk, engaging in activities that promote body confidence, or seeking out role models or mentors who have overcome similar challenges.

4. Building support networks: Connecting individuals with folliculitis to others who share similar experiences can provide a sense of community and reduce feelings of isolation. This may involve facilitating support groups, online forums, or mentorship programs.

By addressing the social stigma and self-esteem issues associated with folliculitis, healthcare providers and patient advocates can help to improve overall quality of life and promote greater understanding and acceptance of individuals with chronic skin conditions.

12.3 Coping Strategies and Support Groups

Living with a chronic skin condition like folliculitis can be challenging, but there are strategies and resources available to help individuals cope with the physical, emotional, and social impacts of the condition. Developing effective coping strategies and seeking out support from others who understand the challenges of living with folliculitis can be key to maintaining overall well-being and quality of life.

12.3.1 Developing a Positive Mindset

One of the most important coping strategies for individuals with folliculitis is to cultivate a positive mindset and focus on the things that are within their control. This may involve:

1. Setting realistic goals: Focusing on achievable goals, such as adhering to a treatment regimen or practicing self-care, can provide a sense of accomplishment and help to maintain motivation.

2. Practicing gratitude: Regularly reflecting on the positive aspects of life, such as supportive relationships or personal strengths, can help to promote a more optimistic outlook.

3. Challenging negative self-talk: Recognizing and challenging negative thoughts or self-talk related to folliculitis can help to reduce their impact on mood and self-esteem.

4. Embracing self-compassion: Treating oneself with kindness and understanding, rather than self-judgment or criticism, can help to promote resilience and emotional well-being.

12.3.2 Engaging in Self-Care Activities

Engaging in regular self-care activities can be an important way to cope with the stress and challenges of living with folliculitis. Some self-care strategies may include:

1. Relaxation techniques: Practicing relaxation techniques, such as deep breathing, progressive muscle relaxation, or mindfulness meditation, can help to reduce stress and promote a sense of calm.

2. Physical activity: Engaging in regular physical activity, such as walking, swimming, or yoga, can help to reduce stress, improve mood, and promote overall health.

3. Hobbies and interests: Pursuing hobbies or interests that bring joy and fulfillment can provide a sense of purpose and help to promote overall well-being.

4. Social connection: Maintaining social connections with friends, family, or support groups can provide a sense of belonging and reduce feelings of isolation.

12.3.3 Seeking Support from Others

Seeking support from others who understand the challenges of living with folliculitis can be a valuable coping strategy. Some sources of support may include:

1. Support groups: Joining a support group for individuals with folliculitis or other chronic skin conditions can provide a sense of community and allow for the sharing of experiences, coping strategies, and resources.

2. Online forums: Participating in online forums or social media groups dedicated to folliculitis can provide a sense of connection and support, particularly for individuals who may not have access to in-person support

groups.

3. Friends and family: Talking with trusted friends or family members about the challenges of living with folliculitis can provide emotional support and help to reduce feelings of isolation.

4. Mental health professionals: Seeking support from a mental health professional, such as a therapist or counselor, can provide a safe and confidential space to process the emotional impact of folliculitis and develop coping strategies.

12.3.4 Advocating for Oneself

Finally, learning to advocate for oneself and one's needs can be an important coping strategy for individuals with folliculitis. This may involve:

1. Communicating with healthcare providers: Regularly communicating with healthcare providers about symptoms, treatment concerns, or emotional well-being can help to ensure that individuals receive the care and support they need.

2. Setting boundaries: Learning to set boundaries around self-care, social activities, or work responsibilities can help to prioritize health and well-being.

3. Seeking accommodations: Advocating for necessary accommodations in work or school settings, such as flexible scheduling or modified dress codes, can help to reduce stress and promote success.

By developing effective coping strategies and seeking out support from others, individuals with folliculitis can build resilience and maintain overall quality of life despite the challenges of living with a chronic skin condition.

12.4 Talking to Your Healthcare Provider

Open and honest communication with healthcare providers is essential for individuals with folliculitis to receive the care and support they need. However, talking about sensitive or personal topics related to skin health can be challenging, particularly if individuals feel self-conscious or embarrassed about their condition. By developing effective communication strategies and building a strong partnership with healthcare providers, individuals with folliculitis can take an active role in their care and work towards optimal management of their condition.

12.4.1 Preparing for Appointments

To make the most of healthcare appointments, it can be helpful for individuals with folliculitis to come prepared with information and questions. This may involve:

1. Keeping a symptom diary: Tracking symptoms, triggers, and treatment responses in a diary or journal can provide valuable information for healthcare providers and help to identify patterns or trends.

2. Making a list of questions: Writing down questions or concerns before the appointment can help to ensure that all important topics are addressed and can provide a useful reference during the visit.

3. Bringing relevant information: Bringing a list of current medications, including over-the-counter products and supplements, can help healthcare providers to identify potential interactions or side effects.

4. Considering bringing a support person: Bringing a trusted friend or family member to the appointment can provide emotional support and help to ensure that important information is not missed.

12.4.2 Discussing Sensitive Topics

Talking about sensitive topics related to folliculitis, such as the impact on self-esteem or sexual functioning, can be challenging but is an important part of receiving comprehensive care. Some strategies for discussing sensitive topics with healthcare providers may include:

1. Being direct and honest: Using clear and direct language to describe symptoms or concerns can help to ensure that healthcare providers have a complete understanding of the situation.

2. Using "I" statements: Using "I" statements, such as "I feel self-conscious about my skin" or "I am concerned about the impact on my relationships," can help to communicate personal experiences and feelings.

3. Asking for clarification: Asking healthcare providers to clarify medical terms or explanations can help to ensure that individuals have a clear understanding of their condition and treatment options.

4. Expressing concerns or fears: Expressing concerns or fears related to folliculitis, such as worries about long-term impact or treatment side effects, can help healthcare providers to provide reassurance and support.

12.4.3 Building a Partnership

Building a strong partnership with healthcare providers is essential for individuals with folliculitis to receive the best possible care. Some strategies for building a partnership may include:

1. Being an active participant: Taking an active role in discussions about diagnosis, treatment options, and management strategies can help to ensure that individuals receive care that aligns with their values and preferences.

2. Following through on recommendations: Following through on recommended treatments or lifestyle modifications can help to demonstrate a commitment to managing folliculitis and can provide valuable feedback for healthcare providers.

3. Communicating concerns or challenges: Communicating any concerns or challenges related to treatment, such as side effects or difficulties with adherence, can help healthcare providers to make necessary adjustments or provide additional support.

4. Expressing gratitude: Expressing gratitude for the care and support provided by healthcare providers can help to build a positive and collaborative relationship.

By developing effective communication strategies and building a strong partnership with healthcare providers, individuals with folliculitis can take an active role in their care and work towards optimal management of their condition.

Conclusion

Folliculitis can have a significant impact on quality of life, affecting individuals physically, emotionally, and socially. From the frustration and disappointment of recurrent outbreaks to the anxiety and self-consciousness that can accompany visible skin lesions, the psychological impact of folliculitis can be profound. Additionally, the social stigma and isolation that can result from visible skin conditions can further compound the negative effects on self-esteem and overall well-being.

To address the multifaceted impact of folliculitis on quality of life, a comprehensive approach that encompasses both medical treatment and emotional support is necessary. Healthcare providers play a critical role in assessing and addressing the psychological and social impact of folliculitis, in addition to providing effective medical management. This may involve screening for mental health concerns, providing education and reassurance, and offering resources for support and coping.

Individuals with folliculitis can also take an active role in managing the impact of their condition on quality of life. Developing effective coping strategies, such as cultivating a positive mindset, engaging in self-care activities, and seeking support from others, can help to build resilience and maintain overall well-being. Additionally, learning to advocate for oneself and one's needs, both with healthcare providers and in social and professional settings, can be an important strategy for managing the challenges of living with a chronic skin condition.

Ultimately, by recognizing the significant impact of folliculitis on quality of life and taking a proactive and comprehensive approach to management, individuals with folliculitis can work towards optimal physical, emotional, and social well-being. Through a strong partnership between healthcare providers and patients, a focus on self-care and coping, and a commitment to reducing stigma and promoting understanding, the negative impact of folliculitis on quality of life can be minimized and individuals can thrive despite the challenges of living with a chronic skin condition.

As we move forward, ongoing research into the psychological and social aspects of folliculitis, as well as the development of new and innovative approaches to management, will be essential. By continuing to advance our understanding of the complex interplay between physical health, mental well-being, and social functioning, we can work towards a future in which individuals with folliculitis are empowered to live their best lives, free from the burden of stigma and limitations imposed by their condition.

CHAPTER 13

Chapter 13: Emerging Therapies and Future Directions

As our understanding of the pathophysiology and management of folliculitis continues to evolve, researchers and clinicians are exploring new and innovative approaches to treatment. From advances in targeted therapies to the development of novel delivery systems, the future of folliculitis management holds promise for more effective, personalized, and convenient care. In this chapter, we will explore some of the emerging therapies and future directions in folliculitis research, including microbiome modulation, targeted immunotherapies, stem cell therapies, and ongoing clinical trials. By staying at the forefront of these advances, healthcare providers can offer their patients the most up-to-date and evidence-based care, while individuals with folliculitis can hold hope for new and improved treatment options on the horizon.

13.1 Microbiome Modulation

The skin microbiome, the complex community of microorganisms that inhabit the skin's surface, has emerged as a key player in the pathogenesis of various skin disorders, including folliculitis. Imbalances in the composition or function of the skin microbiome, known as dysbiosis, have been implicated in the development and exacerbation of folliculitis. As such, strategies aimed at modulating the skin microbiome have garnered significant interest as potential therapeutic approaches for folliculitis.

13.1.1 Probiotics and Prebiotics

Probiotics, live microorganisms that confer health benefits when administered in adequate amounts, have shown promise in the management of various skin conditions, including acne and atopic dermatitis. The use of probiotics in folliculitis is based on the premise that introducing beneficial bacteria to the skin's surface can help to restore a healthy microbiome and prevent the overgrowth of pathogenic organisms. Topical probiotics containing strains of Lactobacillus or Bifidobacterium have been investigated for their potential to reduce inflammation and improve skin barrier function in individuals with folliculitis.

Prebiotics, non-digestible compounds that promote the growth and activity of beneficial bacteria in the gut or on the skin, have also been explored as potential adjuncts to folliculitis treatment. Topical prebiotics, such as certain sugars or plant extracts, may help to selectively promote the growth of beneficial skin bacteria while inhibiting the growth of pathogenic organisms.

13.1.2 Postbiotics and Bacteriophages

Postbiotics, the bioactive compounds produced by probiotic bacteria, have also shown promise in the management of skin disorders. These compounds, which include short-chain fatty acids, peptides, and enzymes, can exert anti-inflammatory, antimicrobial, and immunomodulatory effects on the skin. Topical postbiotics, such as those derived from Lactobacillus or Bifidobacterium, have been investigated for their potential to reduce inflammation and improve skin barrier function in individuals with folliculitis.

Bacteriophages, viruses that specifically infect and kill bacteria, have also emerged as potential tools for modulating the skin microbiome. Phage therapy, the use of bacteriophages to treat bacterial infections, has gained renewed interest in recent years as a potential alternative to antibiotics in the face of increasing antibiotic resistance. In the context of folliculitis, bacteriophages targeting specific pathogenic bacteria, such as Staphylococcus aureus or Pseudomonas aeruginosa, could potentially be used to selectively eliminate these organisms while preserving the beneficial bacteria of the skin microbiome.

13.1.3 Challenges and Future Directions

While microbiome modulation holds promise as a potential therapeutic approach for folliculitis, there are several challenges and limitations to consider. The complex and dynamic nature of the skin microbiome, as well as individual variations in microbiome composition, may make it difficult to develop a one-size-fits-all approach to microbiome modulation. Additionally, the long-term safety and efficacy of probiotics, prebiotics, postbiotics, and bacteriophages in the context of folliculitis management have yet to be fully established.

Future research in this area will need to focus on identifying the specific microbial imbalances associated with different types of folliculitis, as well as developing targeted microbiome modulation strategies that are safe, effective, and personalized to individual patient needs. Larger, well-controlled clinical trials will be necessary to establish the efficacy and safety of these approaches in the management of folliculitis.

13.2 Targeted Immunotherapies

Immunotherapies, treatments that harness the power of the immune system to fight disease, have revolutionized the management of various cancers and autoimmune disorders in recent years. In the context of folliculitis, targeted immunotherapies that modulate specific immune pathways or cytokines involved in the pathogenesis of the condition have shown promise as potential treatment options.

13.2.1 Cytokine Inhibitors

Cytokines, small proteins that regulate immune responses and inflammatory processes, have been implicated in the development and perpetuation of various types of folliculitis. Specific cytokines, such as interleukin (IL)-1, IL-17, and tumor necrosis factor (TNF)-alpha, have been shown to be elevated in the skin of individuals with folliculitis and are thought to contribute to the inflammation and tissue damage associated with the condition.

Cytokine inhibitors, monoclonal antibodies or small molecules that selectively block the action of specific cytokines, have emerged as potential targeted therapies for folliculitis. For example, IL-1 receptor antagonists, such as anakinra, have been investigated for their potential to reduce inflammation and improve symptoms in individuals with neutrophilic folliculitis. Similarly, IL-17 inhibitors, such as secukinumab or ixekizumab, have shown promise in the treatment of pustular psoriasis and hidradenitis suppurativa, conditions that share some pathogenic features with folliculitis.

13.2.2 Janus Kinase Inhibitors

Janus kinase (JAK) inhibitors, small molecule drugs that block the activity of JAK enzymes involved in cytokine signaling, have also emerged as potential targeted therapies for folliculitis. JAK inhibitors, such as tofacitinib and baricitinib, have been shown to modulate the production and activity of various cytokines involved in the pathogenesis of inflammatory skin disorders, including IL-23, IL-17, and interferon-gamma.

In the context of folliculitis, JAK inhibitors have been investigated for their potential to reduce inflammation and improve symptoms in individuals with eosinophilic folliculitis and folliculitis decalvans. Topical formulations of JAK inhibitors have also been developed and are being investigated for their potential to provide localized anti-inflammatory effects while minimizing systemic exposure and side effects.

13.2.3 Challenges and Future Directions

While targeted immunotherapies hold promise as potential treatment options for folliculitis, there are several challenges and limitations to consider. The complex and multifactorial nature of folliculitis pathogenesis, as well as individual variations in immune responses, may make it difficult to develop a one-size-fits-all approach to immunomodulation. Additionally, the long-term safety and efficacy of cytokine inhibitors and JAK inhibitors in the context of folliculitis management have yet to be fully established, particularly in terms of potential side effects and risks associated with long-term immunosuppression.

Future research in this area will need to focus on identifying the specific immune pathways and cytokines involved in different types of folliculitis, as well as developing targeted immunotherapies that are safe, effective, and personalized to individual patient needs. Larger, well-controlled clinical trials will be necessary to establish the efficacy and safety of these approaches in the management of folliculitis, as well as to determine the optimal dosing, duration, and combination of therapies.

13.3 Stem Cell Therapies

Stem cell therapies, treatments that harness the regenerative potential of stem cells to repair or replace damaged tissues, have emerged as a promising approach to the management of various skin disorders, including folliculitis. In the context of folliculitis, stem cell therapies aim to promote the regeneration of damaged hair follicles and surrounding skin, as well as to modulate the inflammatory and immune responses that contribute to the pathogenesis of the condition.

13.3.1 Mesenchymal Stem Cells

Mesenchymal stem cells (MSCs), multipotent adult stem cells that can differentiate into various cell types, including skin and hair follicle cells, have shown promise as potential therapeutic agents for folliculitis. MSCs can be derived from various sources, including bone marrow, adipose tissue, and umbilical cord blood, and have been shown to possess potent immunomodulatory and anti-inflammatory properties.

In the context of folliculitis, MSCs have been investigated for their potential to promote hair follicle regeneration, reduce inflammation, and improve skin barrier function. Preclinical studies have demonstrated that MSCs can migrate to sites of skin inflammation and damage, where they can secrete various growth factors and cytokines that promote tissue repair and regeneration. Additionally, MSCs have been shown to modulate the activity of various immune cells, including T cells and macrophages, which may help to reduce the inflammation and tissue damage associated with folliculitis.

13.3.2 Hair Follicle Stem Cells

Hair follicle stem cells (HFSCs), a population of stem cells that reside in the bulge region of the hair follicle and are responsible for hair follicle regeneration and cycling, have also emerged as potential therapeutic targets for folliculitis. In the context of folliculitis, damage to the hair follicle and surrounding skin can lead to a depletion of HFSCs and impaired hair follicle regeneration, resulting in scarring and permanent hair loss.

Strategies aimed at replenishing or activating HFSCs have been investigated as potential approaches to promoting hair follicle regeneration and reducing scarring in individuals with folliculitis. For example, the transplantation of autologous HFSCs, derived from unaffected areas of the scalp, has been investigated as a potential treatment for scarring folliculitis, such as folliculitis decalvans. Additionally, the use of small molecule drugs or growth factors that target specific pathways involved in HFSC activation and differentiation, such as the Wnt or Shh pathways, has been explored as a potential approach to promoting hair follicle regeneration in the context of folliculitis.

13.3.3 Challenges and Future Directions

While stem cell therapies hold promise as potential treatment options for folliculitis, there are several challenges and limitations to consider. The complex and multifactorial nature of folliculitis pathogenesis, as well as individual variations in stem cell function and regenerative capacity, may make it difficult to develop a one-size-fits-all approach to stem cell therapy. Additionally, the long-term safety and efficacy of stem cell therapies in the context of folliculitis management have yet to be fully established, particularly in terms of potential side effects and risks associated with cell transplantation or manipulation.

Future research in this area will need to focus on identifying the specific stem cell populations and pathways involved in different types of folliculitis, as well as developing targeted stem cell therapies that are safe, effective, and personalized to individual patient needs. Larger, well-controlled clinical trials will be necessary to establish the efficacy and safety of these approaches in the management of folliculitis, as well as to determine the optimal sources, doses, and routes of administration for stem cell therapies. Additionally, efforts to develop standardized protocols and quality control measures for stem cell isolation, expansion, and delivery will be critical to ensuring the reproducibility and reliability of these therapies.

13.4 Ongoing Research and Clinical Trials

As the field of folliculitis research continues to evolve, numerous ongoing studies and clinical trials are investigating novel therapeutic approaches and seeking to refine existing management strategies. These efforts span a wide range of areas, from basic science investigations into the pathophysiology of folliculitis to large-scale clinical trials of new and emerging therapies.

Some examples of ongoing research and clinical trials in the field of folliculitis include:

1. Microbiome studies: Investigators are using advanced sequencing

technologies and bioinformatics tools to characterize the skin microbiome in individuals with different types of folliculitis, with the goal of identifying specific microbial signatures or imbalances that may contribute to the pathogenesis of the condition. These studies may inform the development of targeted microbiome modulation strategies or probiotic therapies for folliculitis.

2. Immunophenotyping studies: Researchers are using flow cytometry, single-cell sequencing, and other advanced techniques to profile the immune cell populations and cytokine networks involved in the pathogenesis of folliculitis. These studies may help to identify novel therapeutic targets or biomarkers for disease activity and treatment response.

3. Targeted therapy trials: Clinical trials are underway to evaluate the safety and efficacy of various targeted therapies for folliculitis, including cytokine inhibitors, JAK inhibitors, and small molecule drugs that target specific pathways involved in inflammation and tissue remodeling. These trials may help to establish the utility of these therapies in the management of different types of folliculitis and inform the development of personalized treatment approaches.

4. Stem cell therapy trials: Investigators are conducting early-phase clinical trials to evaluate the safety and feasibility of stem cell therapies for folliculitis, including the use of autologous MSCs or HFSCs for the treatment of scarring folliculitis. These trials may provide initial proof-of-concept for the use of stem cell therapies in the management of folliculitis and guide the design of larger, randomized controlled trials.

5. Comparative effectiveness studies: Researchers are conducting head-to-head comparisons of different treatment modalities for folliculitis, including topical and systemic therapies, light and laser therapies, and surgical interventions. These studies may help to establish the relative efficacy and safety of different approaches and inform the development of evidence-based

treatment guidelines.

6. Patient-reported outcome studies: Investigators are using validated questionnaires and other patient-reported outcome measures to assess the impact of folliculitis and its treatment on quality of life, psychosocial functioning, and treatment satisfaction. These studies may help to identify the most important outcomes for patients with folliculitis and guide the development of patient-centered care strategies.

As these and other studies continue to advance our understanding of folliculitis and its management, healthcare providers and patients alike can look forward to a future of more personalized, effective, and evidence-based care for this challenging condition. By staying informed about the latest research developments and participating in clinical trials when appropriate, individuals with folliculitis can play an active role in shaping the future of folliculitis management and improving outcomes for themselves and others affected by this condition.

Conclusion

The field of folliculitis research is rapidly evolving, with numerous emerging therapies and future directions holding promise for more effective, personalized, and evidence-based care. From microbiome modulation and targeted immunotherapies to stem cell therapies and ongoing clinical trials, researchers and clinicians are exploring a wide range of innovative approaches to the management of this challenging condition.

As our understanding of the complex pathophysiology of folliculitis continues to deepen, so too does our appreciation of the multifactorial nature of this condition and the need for individualized, multidisciplinary care. By integrating insights from basic science research, translational studies, and clinical trials, healthcare providers can develop more targeted, mechanism-based treatment strategies that address the underlying drivers of folliculitis in each individual patient.

At the same time, the increasing emphasis on patient-reported outcomes and quality of life in folliculitis research underscores the importance of patient-centered care and shared decision-making in the management of this condition. By actively engaging patients in the research process and incorporating their perspectives and priorities into the design and implementation of clinical trials, investigators can ensure that the most meaningful and relevant outcomes are being measured and that the results of these studies are translatable to real-world clinical practice.

Ultimately, the future of folliculitis management will require a collaborative, multidisciplinary approach that brings together researchers, clinicians, patients, and other stakeholders to advance the science and practice of this field. By working together to identify key research priorities, develop innovative therapeutic strategies, and translate research findings into clinical care, we can accelerate progress toward more effective, personalized, and patient-centered management of folliculitis.

As individuals affected by folliculitis, healthcare providers, and researchers, we all have a role to play in shaping the future of this field. By staying informed about the latest research developments, participating in clinical trials when appropriate, and advocating for increased funding and support for folliculitis research, we can help to drive progress and improve outcomes for the millions of individuals worldwide who are affected by this condition. With continued advances in our understanding of the pathophysiology and management of folliculitis, we can look forward to a future in which this once-challenging condition becomes a treatable and manageable aspect of overall skin health and quality of life.

CHAPTER 14

hapter 14: Living Well with Folliculitis: A Comprehensive Guide

Living with folliculitis can be a challenging and often frustrating experience, but with the right knowledge, tools, and support, it is possible to manage this condition effectively and maintain a high quality of life. In this final chapter, we will bring together the key insights and strategies from throughout this book to provide a comprehensive guide to living well with folliculitis. From developing a personalized treatment plan and optimizing nutrition and lifestyle factors to managing stress and building a strong support network, we will explore the multiple dimensions of folliculitis management and provide practical tips and resources for empowering individuals to take control of their skin health and overall well-being.

14.1 Developing a Personalized Treatment Plan

One of the most important aspects of living well with folliculitis is developing a personalized treatment plan that takes into account your unique needs, preferences, and responses to therapy. This process should be a collaborative effort between you and your healthcare provider, with ongoing communication and adjustments as needed to ensure optimal outcomes.

Some key steps in developing a personalized treatment plan for folliculitis include:

1. Identifying your specific type and severity of folliculitis, as well as any potential underlying causes or triggers, through a comprehensive medical evaluation and diagnostic testing as needed.

2. Discussing the potential benefits, risks, and limitations of different treatment options, including topical and systemic therapies, light and laser therapies, and emerging or experimental approaches, and selecting the most appropriate interventions based on your individual goals and preferences.

3. Establishing realistic expectations for treatment outcomes and timelines, and setting clear benchmarks for monitoring progress and adjusting therapy as needed based on your response and any side effects or complications.

4. Incorporating non-pharmacologic strategies for managing folliculitis and optimizing skin health, such as gentle skincare practices, sun protection, and lifestyle modifications, as an integral part of your overall treatment plan.

5. Regularly reviewing and updating your treatment plan in partnership with your healthcare provider, taking into account any changes in your symptoms, quality of life, or overall health status over time.

By taking an active role in developing and implementing your personalized treatment plan, you can ensure that your unique needs and goals are being met and that you are receiving the most effective and appropriate care for your individual situation.

14.2 Nutrition and Diet for Healthy Skin

In addition to medical therapies, nutrition and diet can play an important role in managing folliculitis and promoting overall skin health. While there is no one-size-fits-all diet for folliculitis, certain dietary patterns and nutrients have been associated with reduced inflammation, improved skin barrier function, and enhanced wound healing, all of which may be beneficial for individuals with this condition.

Some key dietary strategies for supporting skin health in the context of folliculitis include:

1. Consuming a balanced, nutrient-dense diet that includes a variety of fruits, vegetables, whole grains, lean proteins, and healthy fats, to provide the essential building blocks for skin repair and regeneration.

2. Ensuring adequate intake of key skin-supporting nutrients, such as vitamin A, vitamin C, vitamin D, vitamin E, zinc, and omega-3 fatty acids, through a combination of dietary sources and targeted supplementation as needed.

3. Limiting consumption of processed, high-glycemic, and pro-inflammatory foods, such as refined carbohydrates, added sugars, and unhealthy fats, which may exacerbate inflammation and impair skin barrier function.

4. Staying well-hydrated by drinking plenty of water and other non-caffeinated, non-alcoholic beverages throughout the day, to support skin moisture and elasticity.

5. Considering potential food triggers or sensitivities that may exacerbate folliculitis symptoms, such as dairy, gluten, or spicy foods, and working with a registered dietitian or nutritionist to identify and eliminate any problematic foods as needed.

It is important to note that while dietary modifications can be a helpful adjunct to medical therapies for folliculitis, they should not be used as a substitute for evidence-based treatments or professional medical advice. Always consult with your healthcare provider before making significant changes to your diet or starting any new supplements, to ensure safety and appropriateness for your individual situation.

14.3 Stress Management Techniques

Stress is a well-known trigger for many skin conditions, including folliculitis, and effective stress management is an essential component of any comprehensive folliculitis management plan. Chronic stress can exacerbate inflammation, impair immune function, and interfere with skin barrier repair, all of which can contribute to the development and persistence of folliculitis lesions.

Fortunately, there are many evidence-based stress management techniques that can help individuals with folliculitis reduce their stress levels, improve their overall well-being, and support optimal skin health. Some effective strategies include:

1. Regular exercise: Engaging in moderate-intensity physical activity, such as brisk walking, cycling, or swimming, for at least 30 minutes per day, most days of the week, can help reduce stress, improve mood, and promote overall health.

2. Mind-body practices: Techniques such as deep breathing, progressive muscle relaxation, meditation, and yoga can help calm the mind, reduce physical tension, and promote a sense of inner peace and well-being.

3. Cognitive-behavioral therapy (CBT): This evidence-based form of psychotherapy can help individuals identify and change negative thought patterns and behaviors that contribute to stress, and develop more adaptive coping strategies.

4. Social support: Building and maintaining a strong network of supportive relationships, whether through family, friends, or support groups, can provide a vital source of emotional support and practical assistance in managing the challenges of living with folliculitis.

5. Healthy lifestyle habits: Adopting healthy lifestyle practices, such as getting adequate sleep, limiting alcohol and caffeine intake, and avoiding smoking and other harmful substances, can help reduce overall stress levels and promote optimal health and well-being.

Incorporating regular stress management practices into your daily routine can help you build resilience, cope more effectively with the challenges of living with folliculitis, and support your overall skin health and quality of life. If you are struggling with chronic stress or anxiety, don't hesitate to seek professional help from a mental health provider who can provide additional guidance and support.

14.4 Empowering Yourself: Advocacy and Education

Finally, one of the most important aspects of living well with folliculitis is empowering yourself through advocacy and education. By taking an active role in your own care, staying informed about the latest research and treatment options, and advocating for your needs and rights as a patient, you can ensure that you are receiving the best possible care and support for managing your condition.

Some key ways to empower yourself as an individual living with folliculitis include:

1. Educating yourself about folliculitis: Take the time to learn about the different types and causes of folliculitis, the available treatment options, and the latest research and clinical trials in this field. This book is a great starting point, but there are also many other reliable sources of information, such as medical journals, patient advocacy organizations, and online support communities.

2. Communicating openly with your healthcare provider: Don't be afraid to ask questions, express your concerns, and provide feedback to your

healthcare provider about your symptoms, treatment progress, and overall quality of life. Remember, you are an equal partner in your care, and your input and perspectives are valuable and important.

3. Advocating for your needs and rights: If you feel that your needs are not being met or that you are not receiving appropriate care for your folliculitis, don't hesitate to speak up and advocate for yourself. This may involve seeking a second opinion, filing a complaint with a regulatory agency, or joining a patient advocacy organization to push for better research, treatment, and support for individuals with folliculitis.

4. Connecting with others: Building connections with other individuals living with folliculitis, whether through online forums, support groups, or patient advocacy organizations, can provide a valuable source of emotional support, practical advice, and collective advocacy. By sharing your experiences and learning from others, you can gain new insights, strategies, and confidence for managing your condition and living your best life.

5. Participating in research: If you are interested and eligible, consider participating in clinical trials or other research studies related to folliculitis. By contributing your time, data, and perspectives, you can help advance scientific understanding of this condition and contribute to the development of new and better treatments for yourself and others living with folliculitis.

By empowering yourself through advocacy and education, you can take control of your folliculitis journey and ensure that you are receiving the best possible care and support for managing this condition and maximizing your overall health and well-being.

Conclusion

Living well with folliculitis requires a comprehensive, multidimensional approach that encompasses personalized treatment planning, optimal nutrition and lifestyle practices, effective stress management, and self-empowerment through advocacy and education. By taking an active role in your own care and working collaboratively with your healthcare provider and support network, you can develop the knowledge, skills, and confidence needed to manage this condition effectively and maintain a high quality of life.

Throughout this book, we have explored the many facets of folliculitis, from its underlying causes and risk factors to the latest advances in diagnosis, treatment, and prevention. We have emphasized the importance of a holistic, patient-centered approach to folliculitis management, one that takes into account the unique needs, preferences, and experiences of each individual living with this condition.

As you continue on your folliculitis journey, remember that you are not alone, and that there is hope and support available to you. By staying informed, advocating for your needs, and connecting with others who understand what you are going through, you can build the resilience, courage, and determination needed to live well with folliculitis and achieve your full potential for health and happiness.

We hope that this book has provided you with valuable insights, strategies, and inspiration for managing your folliculitis and optimizing your overall well-being. Remember, your skin health is an integral part of your overall health, and by taking proactive steps to care for your skin and your whole self, you can unlock your innate capacity for healing, growth, and vitality.

As the field of folliculitis research and care continues to evolve, stay curious, stay engaged, and stay committed to your own health and well-being. Together, we can create a brighter, healthier, and more hopeful future for all those living with folliculitis, one day at a time.

CONCLUSION

Throughout this comprehensive guide, we have explored the multifaceted nature of folliculitis, a common yet often misunderstood skin condition that affects millions of people worldwide. From its underlying causes and risk factors to the latest advances in diagnosis, treatment, and prevention, we have sought to provide a holistic, evidence-based approach to understanding and managing this complex condition.

At the heart of this book is the recognition that folliculitis is not just a physical condition, but one that can have profound impacts on an individual's emotional, social, and overall well-being. We have emphasized the importance of a patient-centered, collaborative approach to folliculitis management, one that takes into account the unique needs, preferences, and experiences of each individual living with this condition.

Beginning with an overview of the different types and presentations of folliculitis, we have provided a foundation for understanding the diverse ways in which this condition can manifest and the key factors that contribute to its development and persistence. We have explored the role of bacterial, fungal, and viral infections, as well as non-infectious factors such as hormonal imbalances, medications, and underlying medical conditions, in the pathogenesis of folliculitis.

Moving on to diagnosis and evaluation, we have highlighted the importance of a thorough, systematic approach to assessing folliculitis, one that combines clinical examination, laboratory testing, and histopathologic analysis as needed to accurately characterize the type and severity of the condition. We have also emphasized the role of differential diagnosis in distinguishing folliculitis from other similar-appearing skin conditions, and the importance of identifying any underlying systemic or contributing factors.

In our discussion of treatment options, we have provided a comprehensive overview of the various medical and non-pharmacologic interventions available for managing folliculitis, from topical and systemic antimicrobials to light and laser therapies, immunomodulators, and emerging targeted therapies. We have emphasized the importance of a personalized, multi-modal approach to treatment, one that takes into account the specific type and severity of folliculitis, as well as individual patient factors such as age, comorbidities, and treatment preferences.

Beyond medical interventions, we have also highlighted the critical role of self-care and lifestyle modifications in managing folliculitis and optimizing overall skin health. From gentle skincare practices and sun protection to stress management, healthy nutrition, and regular exercise, we have provided practical tips and strategies for supporting skin barrier function, reducing inflammation, and promoting wound healing.

Recognizing the significant impact that folliculitis can have on quality of life, we have dedicated a chapter to exploring the emotional, social, and psychological dimensions of living with this condition. We have discussed the challenges of coping with chronic, recurrent skin lesions, the stigma and self-consciousness that can accompany visible skin conditions, and the importance of building a strong support network and advocating for one's needs and rights as a patient.

Looking to the future, we have provided an overview of the exciting emerging therapies and research directions in the field of folliculitis, from microbiome modulation and targeted immunotherapies to stem cell therapies and personalized medicine approaches. We have emphasized the importance of ongoing research and clinical trials in advancing our understanding of this complex condition and developing new and better treatments for those affected.

Perhaps most importantly, we have sought to empower individuals living with folliculitis to take an active role in their own care and well-being. By providing a comprehensive, accessible guide to understanding and managing this condition, we hope to equip readers with the knowledge, tools, and strategies needed to navigate their folliculitis journey with confidence and resilience.

As we conclude this book, we want to remind readers that living well with folliculitis is possible, and that there is hope and support available. By staying informed, advocating for their needs, and connecting with others who understand their experiences, individuals with folliculitis can build the skills and confidence needed to manage this condition effectively and maintain a high quality of life.

We also want to emphasize the importance of continued research, education, and advocacy in the field of folliculitis. By working together to advance scientific understanding, develop new and better treatments, and raise awareness and support for those affected, we can create a brighter, healthier, and more hopeful future for all those living with this condition.

To the healthcare providers, researchers, and other professionals working in the field of folliculitis, we urge you to continue your dedicated efforts to improve the care and outcomes for those affected. By staying up-to-date with the latest research and best practices, collaborating across disciplines and specialties, and prioritizing patient-centered, compassionate care, you can make a meaningful difference in the lives of those you serve.

And to the individuals living with folliculitis, we want to leave you with a message of hope and encouragement. Your skin health is an integral part of your overall health and well-being, and you deserve access to the best possible care and support for managing this condition. Remember that you are not alone, and that there are resources and communities available to help you along your journey.

By taking proactive steps to care for your skin and your whole self, seeking out the support and guidance you need, and advocating for your needs and rights as a patient, you can unlock your innate capacity for healing, resilience, and vitality. Trust in your own strength and wisdom, and know that a fulfilling, vibrant life is possible, even in the face of the challenges of living with folliculitis.

As we close this book, we want to express our deep gratitude to all those who have contributed to our understanding and management of folliculitis, from the researchers and clinicians who have dedicated their careers to this field, to the patients and advocates who have shared their stories and perspectives. It is through your collective efforts and insights that we have been able to compile this comprehensive guide, and it is through your ongoing dedication and collaboration that we will continue to make progress in the fight against folliculitis.

So let us move forward together, with renewed commitment, compassion, and hope, in the pursuit of better health, well-being, and quality of life for all those affected by folliculitis. May this book serve as a valuable resource and companion on your journey, and may you find the strength, support, and inspiration you need to live well with folliculitis, one day at a time.